Trouble With The Man Gland

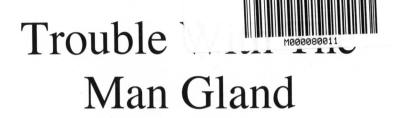

Journeys Of a Scientist Patient Exploring The Science of Advanced Prostate Cancer

Otto F. Sankey, Ph.D.

Published by Schwarz Publishing House

All Rights Reserved. No part of this book may be reproduced, scanned, or distributed in any printed or electronic form without permission.

ISBN 978-0-9961319-4-0

Printed in the United States of America.
Date of First Printing, August, 2015
10 9 8 7 6 5 4 3 2 1

Disclaimer

The material in this book is NOT MEDICAL ADVICE. The information is to be used for educational and informational purposes only. The author is a scientist, not a licensed medical professional. For medical treatment, diagnosis or the use of drugs, a qualified medical professional must always be consulted. The opinions expressed herein are those of the author, and not necessarily the publisher, and may or may not be shared by others in the medical, scientific, and/or patient community. Scientific opinions can and do change with time, and experiments are always subject to interpretation.

A serious effort was made to provide accurate information, but the author or the publisher makes no guarantee. Warnings about drugs, therapies, and procedures are either incomplete or are not given, and their presence or absence does not indicate that they are safe, effective, or appropriate.

Credits
Most diagrams and biological schematics created by Otto F. Sankey
Figure manipulation, GIMP (GNU Image Manipulation Program) www.gimp.org
Protein ribbon figures made with Jmol software, an open-source Java viewer for chemical structures in 3D.
http://www.jmol.org/
Biological components from Servier Medical Art Slide kits, http://servier.com/Powerpoint-image-bank, Licensed under creative commons attribution, creativecommons.org/licenses/by/3.0/
Public domain clipart courtesy http://openclipart.org

Diagram of the neighborhood of the prostate, Courtesy, National Cancer Institute, Alan Hoofring (Illustrator).

Microtubules during cell division. National Heart, Lung, and Blood Institute, National Institutes of Health, Creator Nasser Rusan.

Cartoon of epithelial cells, Frontiers of Oncology 3, Article 273 (2013), Disruption of prostate epithelial differentiation pathways and prostate cancer evelopment, SB Frank and CK Miranti. Courtesy Prof. Miranti.

Cover figures
Prostate cells showing Adenocarcinoma, Courtesy, CDC Dr Edwin P. Ewing,Jr., Pubic Health Image Library (PHIL)
Sky Blue Prostate Cancer , Ribbon, Courtesy public domain clipart, openclipart.org

Cover Design: Frank J. Fister

DEDICATION

This book is dedicated to Debra A. Sankey, my spouse of over 40 years. She has been with me through this incredible journey called life and raising a family. She is my personal Mother Teresa.

vi

ACKNOWLEDGMENTS

Thanks to my family, spouse Debra and children Holly, Robyn and Stephanie for offering complete support while writing this book, during treatment of this disease, and putting up with a scientist who spent much of his time at work following his dream.

I am indebted to my physician team who is treating me including oncologists Dr Christopher Kellogg, Dr. Steven Finkelstein, and Dr. Mark Scholz, and urologist Dr. David Grossklaus. Together we made a Lewis and Clark Corps of Discovery for this journey of mine. Thanks to Frank Fister for his expertise creating the covers and ironing out some problems with figures. Thanks to Stephanie Sankey for showing me some of the tips and tricks concerning publishing. Also thanks to Kelly Huey for advancing our UsTOO prostate Cancer Support Group. Finally, thanks to my copy editor, Kathy Williamson

Table of contents

Trouble With The Man Gland

Otto F. Sankey, Ph.D.

Preface

We are drowning in information, while starving for wisdom. The world henceforth will be run by synthesizers, people able to put together the right information at the right time, think critically about it, and make important choices wisely. E.O Wilson, American biologist/naturalist.

Although it is the most frequently diagnosed cancer in men, prostate cancer is highly misunderstood. The disease has little effect on many, yet it is deadly to others. The book is a form of expedition—an expedition to explore the scientific wildernesses of biology, chemistry, and physics of the mechanisms that promote and fuel the deadly form of the Prostate Cancer. We journey through the modern understanding of the disease that physicians use to exploit its weaknesses, and that result in therapies to reduce or mitigate its devastation.

The expedition is for those who want to dig deeper into the subject. The account is written in understandable terms for a layman, yet retains some scientific rigor without the numbing jargon used in evidence-based scientific and medical journals. The terrain covered is not the initial treatments of prostate cancer—watchful waiting or active surveillance, proton therapy, brachytherapy, external beam therapy, or radical prostatectomy. There are many good books on these topics. This book is primarily about when prostate cancer takes a turn for the worse, and becomes advanced. Most books stop, or say little, on this topic. We pop the hood and take a look at the inner workings of the disease—the science of the disease, its weak points that therapies attempt to exploit, and we examine some of the experiments that got us to our current understanding. This kind of information is difficult to find in an easily digestible form. Books are less likely to be found on these topics as it is not "mass market," and frankly is much more difficult to write. Hundreds of scientific papers have to be researched to keep up with developments. It should appeal to those with the curiosity of a cat, or the inquisitiveness of a scientist.

The magic of several beautiful experiments is explained. As such, prostate cancer patients, scientists, engineers, and biotechnologists who want to get an overview of the science applied to this important health menace will benefit from the expedition.

Advanced prostate cancer is a disease that must be fought, and fought hard. Like a military fight, its afflicted must become warriors against the disease. Part of the war chest of a warrior is intelligence (information). As EO Wilson tells us above, we need information to synthesize if we are to produce wisdom. And an abundance of wisdom (and luck) is needed to be successful in the fight. It is not just a patient's physicians that lead the prostate cancer journey that a prostate cancer warrior takes, but instead it is a partnership between patient and physician. The expedition for the reader results in providing current information about the science of the disease so that the prostate cancer warrior becomes a kind of Captain Clark, who works side by side with his co-expedition physician leader Captain Lewis to explore the forbidding landscape of this disease. Upriver, we go!

Chapter 1

Watch Out For trouble.

Life is what happens while you are busy making other plans.
John Lennon

Prostate cancer is very slow growing, except when it isn't. The slow growth causes many men to put it out of their minds. After all, we can't face the fact that there is a problem "down there." It goes to a man's core. Many troubles with the prostate remain indolent, meaning they can remain in that state for many years and not cause problems. But prostate cancer is unfortunately all too common, and for the unlucky few with the aggressive variety that develops into advanced prostate cancer it is a life-changing, life-shortening, event. Those with advanced prostate cancer create a modified **Credo** for life—live a more meaningful life, protect your quality of life and become a warrior advocate for your case. Becoming a warrior includes being knowledgeable of the disease and doing what it takes to live long enough to die of something else before prostate cancer (PCa) gets you.

The prostate is not needed to lead a healthy life, at least late in life when the prostate causes trouble. Men in their 60s and 70s are usually no longer siring children, although they desire to go through the motions with gusto. Men with *localized* prostate cancer often have their prostate removed surgically, a procedure called a radical prostatectomy. This is just one of many ways to treat localized prostate cancer.

The word localized should not go unnoticed, as it should be shouting out. If the disease is confined locally in the prostate, the chances for a complete enduring cure are very high. Most of the discussion about prostate cancer is about what to do when it is localized and what events to worry about that could happen.

Surgery or many different forms of radiation can be used when it is localized. Those who have gotten one specific treatment will argue with conviction that it worked for them and if your case is like theirs (likely it is not), it will work for you too. However, nothing is 100% and a significant fraction of treated patients relapse and progress to advanced disease and metastasis (spread) to other parts of the body.

The source of the trouble is the prostate gland, a sexual gland the size of a walnut, about 3-4 cm in its normal state. It is in the neighborhood of prime real estate. (**See Figure 1-1**) It is located below the bladder, in front of the rectum, and in back of the pelvis. The urethra from the bladder and the seminal vesicles from the testis run through it to the penis. The prostate secretes

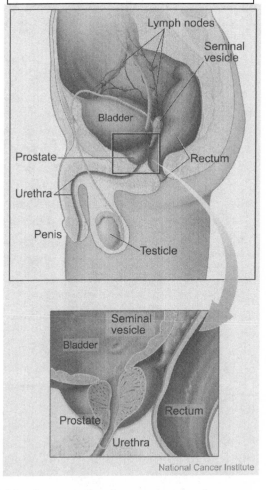

Figure 1-1. From the National Cancer Institute, Alan Hoofring.

seminal fluids to aid in the reproductive process and may provide spermal nutrients. The fluid state of semen is aided by prostate specific antigen (PSA), a protease enzyme that can cut up proteins to better make semen fluid.

Metastasis is the watershed event. The trouble that prostate cancer produces when it moves to other parts of the body is a new degree of Trouble. Trouble with a capital T. The patient is no longer a cancer survivor, but is surviving cancer. Like in a delicate negotiation, the negotiators have pounded their fists on the table have left in a huff. There is no turning back the clock or second chances. When cancer is localized in the prostate it is still curable. When metastasized, a full cure is not possible. It becomes important to remember the Credo and fight to lead a meaningful quality of life and to die naturally of something else before you die of prostate cancer.

How does the watershed event of metastasis take place? Cancer is a heterogeneous disease—not all the cancer cells are the same. In the prostate gland there often are different clones of cells that have gone awry to produce the cancer. Each clone produces a colony, and each clone has its own genetic signature and starts at a certain spot. The different clones likely appeared at different times, all building up to produce the primary cancer within the prostate. But metastasis is different. Research in 2009 at Johns Hopkins has shown (by studying copy number variations in DNA) that in most, and possibly all cases, there is a single initial cancer cell that produces most metastases. This means that metastasis lesions have a common origin and perhaps came from a single escaping cell that established itself elsewhere then proliferated. It is estimated that there are 3.7×10^{13} (that's about 40 trillion) cells in a human body. A few become cancerous, and perhaps one metastasizes and escapes the prostate and finds a comfortable home in the bone or lymph nodes. It is amazing the Trouble an aggressive single cell can cause.

The situation is reminiscent of terrorism. A few miscreants wreak havoc on an entire country. And they hide effectively. That is why men who have "taken care" of their cancer must always be on the alert. A few cells remaining in

4

a "sleeper cell" can awaken producing a small metastatic lesion. Initially they are too small to detect, and often we are made aware of their presence by an increase of PSA blood serum levels.

Our Expedition

This is an undertaking fraited (sic, freighted) with many difficulties. But my friend, I do assure you that no man lives with whom I would prefer to undertake such a trip as yourself. Wm Clark to Meriwether Lewis, 1803

An expedition will take place on these pages and you are invited along. Our orders are to explore the advanced and metastatic prostate cancer landscape. Our journey will be like that of Lewis and Clark. We will be exploring the advanced metastatic prostate landscape with an eye to unveiling the science of how prostate cancer works, and how therapies are trying to take advantage of this science. We will examine therapies that are both FDA approved and therapies that are not. The Lewis and Clark Corps of Discovery did not know what they were going to find. Some suggested they would encounter mastodons, as skeletons were found near Philadelphia in 1801, and perhaps living ancestors were still alive in the West. Metastatic prostate cancer is similarly unchartered, with many questions and few answers. There are often several contradicting answers to a single question allowing many maps to be made and to follow in order to produce a successful advance.

Investigating the science along the journey produces hope. There have been advances in recent years, but we are still waiting for that game-changing advance. The problem is difficult but it is not that difficult. (Sorry, that was too easy to say.) Once the "answer" is known, it all will seem so obvious. Science builds as a snowball—one advance produces another, then another and so on. Right now our snowball is still small but that next patch of snowball building snow may exist in the science literature right now. As E.O. Wilson tells us in the preface, *"The world henceforth will be run by synthesizers, people able to put together the right information at the right time, think critically about it, and make important choices wisely."*

The expedition will not be easy. It is not light reading because it is not a light subject. An attempt is made to take the complexities of Prostate Cancer (PCa) science and make it understandable. Lewis and Clark found trouble all along the way, including a life threatening winter. They had to travel upstream along the Missouri River, and that was the easy part. We too will be going upstream, moving against the often-numbing difficulty that PCa science will present to us. The reading at times will be like fighting the current, but try to hang in and not let the river take you down. I'll try to keep the jargon down to a minimum. Hopefully the reward is that you will begin to understand the science of advanced prostate cancer and its therapies and also see that the science offers hope. Eventually the Lewis and Clark expedition made it triumphantly to the Pacific Ocean, but they had to work for it.

This chapter is an introduction, and will continue with the generalities of prostate cancer. We are picking up provisions at the confluence of the Missouri and Mississippi Rivers, preparing to soon head up the mighty Missouri.

My story

My personal case is typical in some aspects and unusual in other aspects. As they say, "No two cases are alike." The story starts when I was 62 years old when I was initially diagnosed. Within 2 months from initial diagnosis, prostate cancer completely changed my life. My diagnosis started as a typical case. The PSA blood test showed a level past the "take notice" levels of 4 or 5ng/dL, specifically my level was 5.6ng/mL. In addition there was some hesitancy with urination during the day and frequent urination at night.

These and the gradual rise over the years in PSA level is a signal to the primary care physician to send you to a Urologist. A digital rectal exam revealed nothing, but my urologist suggested a tissue biopsy—a transrectal ultrasound

(TRUS) guided biopsy. Ultrasound is used to image the prostate to help guide the 12 (or so) needles that take tissue samples. No one wants to have that done, but of course I did have it performed. Although not a pleasant procedure, it was fairly uneventful. The worst of it is getting the instrument into your rectum, and some bleeding afterwards which required a pad. I had gone through life until this point with no health problems at all. Exercise was always in my weekly agenda, and as I retired 2 years earlier, gym visits occurred usually three times per week. I took many of the classes— Zumba, body pump, yoga, and complete-fitness. So a TRUS biopsy was fairly big, and unusual, event for me.

A pathologist examines the tissue from a biopsy, and the result came back as a Gleason 6 prostate cancer. Gleason 6 is a fairly low grade of prostate cancer, and there are those who even wish to call it something else besides cancer. Here's the rub to this situation. Biopsies are a hit and miss procedure. If they find something, it likely is true (few false positives). But if they don't find anything, it does not mean you are whole—there are false negatives. My view now is that whatever the result of a biopsy is, your situation is that or worse.

Next came the first phase of my education about prostate cancer. The urologist explained the alternatives in a nutshell fashion, but my main education came from reading some of the many books available on treatments after initial diagnosis. The general advice that I received was the younger you are and the healthier you are, the more aggressive you should be concerning your treatment. I felt in excellent health, and at 62 was still relatively young. After all, the Beatles indicated that a senior life only begins "When I'm sixty-four."

I decided on robot assisted laparoscopic surgery (Da Vinci) to remove the prostate—a radical prostatectomy. The concept was that if the cancer were entirely localized within the prostate, this would in fact be as close to a "cure" as one could hope. The surgery required an anesthesia and is a serious affair, but it all went well. No cancer was found in the margins, and there were no signs of cancer on adjacent lymph nodes. There were one-inch incisions several places on the abdomen with the largest being above the navel. After the surgery, a catheter in the urethra had to be worn for 2 weeks, which I found to be the worst part of the affair. I have a laboratory chemistry stand in my small home laboratory that I adjusted to hold the urine bag. For that two weeks, I never left the house, was in pajamas and a robe, and watched the complete set of episodes of "You Bet Your Life" with Groucho Marx from the 50s-60s on Netflix. Groucho would have had a blast interviewing me in my PJs with my trusty urine bag hanging from a test tube clamp. Things were not looking bright, but I did push through for the two weeks.

Shortly thereafter, a series of bad news flashes were received. One has to wait a month or more to recheck your PSA after a prostatectomy. Finally upon rechecking the PSA level, it was found not to be low, but higher than when I started. A couple of retries of the PSA blood test to be sure showed that the PSA level was ever increasing—reaching 44ng/mL. Recall before surgery the level was 5.6ng/mL. One is expected to have a very low PSA, and ultimately an undetectable one, after a prostatectomy. Where is prostate specific antigen coming from if you do not have a prostate? Clearly something is amiss.

The second bit of bad news came with the pathologist report on the tissue of the prostate itself. Since it is out of the body, a complete analysis can be performed, far more than the limited hit or miss sampling of a biopsy. The pathologist report showed it was Gleason 10, not Gleason 6 as found in the biopsy. Gleason 10 means the prostate cells are undifferentiated or little so—it no longer is going to act like a prostate cell, but is in a very aggressive cancerous state.

Based on the rising PSA, the urologist ordered a Technetium 99(metastable) bone scan. This is the typical bone scan used to determine if there is metastasis of prostate cancer to the bone. It indicated that I had many lesion of cancer on the bone. This is of course the devastating news we did not want to hear. The one bit of good news was that

MRI showed now evidence of internal organ metastasis. This was unexpected good news, as at the time it seemed that the each bit of news was worse than the one before.

In a period of a couple of months I had gone from an apparently healthy individual, to one with a fairly low but concerning PSA, to signs of a confirmed but not very aggressive cancer, to a patient with metastatic stage 4 advanced prostate cancer disease. The stakes became extremely high. That is when I transformed myself into a prostate cancer warrior. I intend to use my background as a scientist to learn everything I can about the disease, and become a prostate cancer fighter and advocate, including writing this book.

The knowledge of the science of prostate cancer helps me (and I hope you too) to form that Lewis and Clark team, of patient and oncologist, as you enter into that unforgiving wilderness of fighting the disease.

Lies, Damned Lies, And Statistics
(Mark Twain)

Life has many perils and PCa is just one of them. But it's important to know your odds so you can lead a life that attempts to minimize some of the perils and escape them, if you are lucky.

Prostate cancer is the most commonly diagnosed cancer in men. Each year 218,000 men are diagnosed with prostate cancer and 32,000 men die from it. Although it is the most frequently diagnosed cancer, lung cancer is the most deadly with 223,000 (men and women) diagnosed and 86,000 deaths.

So what are your chances of dying from prostate cancer? Currently there are 299,000 male deaths from cancer in the US each year, so PCa accounts for only about 11%, while Lung cancer accounts for about 35% of male cancer deaths. Of course, smoking is a large contributor to lung cancer. A health-minded individual can lower his odds by never smoking. But there is not much you can do about prostate cancer, except try to live in a clean healthy environment, eat well, exercise, and hope that it all makes a difference.

When we look at overall numbers in all age groups, cardiovascular disease (CVD) is the number one killer with a chance of dying from CVD of about 24%, with cancer not far behind at 23%. The bottom line concerning PCa for men is this — 1 in about 35 men will die because of prostate cancer. I visualize a classroom of (male) students. Upper level college classes are often of this size. One student of a male only class (that must be one of my physics classes) will be destined to die of prostate cancer. It's not nearly as deadly as CVD where one in four will die. Perhaps that is again one of the reasons symptoms of PCa are often ignored. We somehow conclude it is not that fatal.

The statistics of prostate cancer diagnosis and mortality are very much like those of a dice game where throwing a "1" gets you into Trouble. Each man gets either one or two throws of a single dice, depending. All men throw at least once, and the first throw determines whether you will ever be diagnosed with prostate cancer. Since the odds of this are one in six, you are safe unless you throw a "1." If you did not throw a "1" you are safe and need not worry about prostate cancer. However if you did throw a "1" you must throw again. This time you are throwing for your life! If it comes up "1" again (another one in six chance), that's snake eyes—unfortunately you lose.

Prostate cancer is even more common than the health statistics show. One way to see when prostate occurs is to study cadavers—specifically those whose death was brought on by other means. Living souls do not want their prostate dissected unless they are sure they have prostate cancer. But cadavers are more willing subjects. A study in 2009 assessed the prostates of 133 male cadavers in Australia. The coroner ordered these autopsies and the subjects had died for any number of reasons. Seventy of were above 50 years of age and 63 were younger than 50.

The high rate of prostate cancer that was found is alarming. Of those over 50 years of age, 21 out of 70 (35%) had prostate cancer while 18 (25.7%) had invasive prostate cancer capable of spreading to other parts of the body. Other studies have found similar results; it is not something peculiar to those down-under Australians. Recent estimates range from 30-70% for those over 60 years of age to have prostate cancer. There is some good news. Of the 63 cadavers that were less than 50 years old, only one had invasive PCa.

It is an older man's disease but ramps up quickly with age, with 60 being a particularly important age. African Americans are more prone to the disease and at an earlier age. But let's not get lost in statistics. The real message is that prostate cancer is not rare. You could have it (if you are male). However, the really aggressive variety, what our expedition is about, is fairly rare. So you can relax... a bit.

Production of Cancer

Cancer occurs when the control pathways within a cell become malfeasant. Cells grow uncontrollably becoming neoplastic (new growth) and produce tumor growths. Cells normally live a communal lifestyle, dying at the appropriate time in a controlled fashion in a process called apoptosis, or programmed cell death, a form of cell suicide. Corruption of the apoptosis pathway allows the cell to live on and the cell loses its sense of communal obligation. It becomes selfish, wanting to live on forever and to reproduce uncontrollably. Knowing this gives us one potential target to win the battle. Restore the apoptosis pathway in these cells without causing other cells to unnecessarily enhance apoptosis, and the cells will kill themselves for you. No need to poison them, and you, with chemotherapy. If only we could figure our exactly how to do this. We can do it in a test tube, but it's not so easily accomplished on a human being.

The cell becomes neoplastic due to mutations in the genes of the cell. Genes become altered so they code incorrectly. Genes are a DNA sequences in the nucleus of a cell that codes for proteins, and proteins are the functioning nano-machines of the body. Alterations of genes change the abundance, content, form and function of the proteins. Luck plays a role. Genetic mutations are often harmless, but sometimes they are not. Prostate cancer is not produced by a single mutation, but by a sequence of mutations. Mutations may occur by chance during gestation, by chance during your lifetime, by chemical or environmental mutagens (blackened beef is often cited as a source of other forms of cancer), and by epigenetics. Epigenetics produces changes in gene expression on top of (epi-) genetics. The need for numerous mutations largely explains why prostate cancer occurs in older men. It takes time for the mutations to accumulate to produce a cancerous cell. The situation is not so black and white however as many mutations make no difference. But there are those in certain genes that are critical for prostate cancer.

Prostate cancer is not just one uniform disease, but it has many "flavors" due to the specific genetic aberrations, the type of cells affected, the genes that are being expressed, and the genes that are being shut down (like those affecting the apoptosis pathway). The disease is complex—if you've seen once case of prostate cancer, you've seen one case of prostate cancer. Even within the same individual, different foci (as specific regions of cancer cell growth are called) may be different on the genetic level. President Obama announced his precision medicine (AKA personalized medicine) initiative in the 2015 State of the Union message, which potentially more precisely diagnoses an individual's cancer and better indicates effective therapies. There has been much research in trying to identify the particular flavor one has of prostate cancer so as not to waste time on administering treatments that will not be effective and are loaded with side effects.

To illustrate the general non-conformity of prostate cancer, let's quantify the kind of variations one may see. A particular experiment, completed in 2013 and led by Knezevic of Genomic Health, looked at the expression of 12 cancer-related genes from cells obtained from prostate cancer needle biopsies. Their end game was to find signatures of indolent (non-aggressive) versus aggressive disease. We can label each of the twelve A, B, ... L. Let's take as an example all patients that had just three (n=3) of these twelve (N=12) genes being highly expressed. There are many variations, as a patient may be expressing ABC, or ABD, ..., or JKL. The number of different variations in this simple example is 220. (For math mavens, this is $N!/(N-n)!n!$, or $12!/(9!3!)=220$.) The point being illustrated is this; no two prostate cancers are alike.

There is a dramatic increase in the incidence of prostate cancer with age. Mathematical models simplistically describe cancer incidence as a power law,

$$I_c = A\ t^p$$

where I_c is the incidence rate of cancer with age, t is the age in years, and p is the power. The parameter "A" is a constant and varies for different cancers. The purpose of mentioning a power law is to illustrate the **dramatic increases** of incidence as age (t) increases. For example for a power p of 8, changing the age from t=40y to t=70y increases the incidence rate I_c by a factor of $(70/40)^8=88$ (that is the ratio of I_c (at 70y) to that of I_c (at 40y)). Such a huge increase in the Incidence rate of prostate cancer is seen in the data shown in the **Table 1-1** ($\sim894/10.5 = 85.1$).

Table 1-1. The incidence rate of *invasive* prostate cancer (2007-2011 data, From the *Seer Cancer Statistics Review 1975-2011*).

(t) Age at diagnosis/death	(I_c) Incidence Rate per 100,000 Individuals
25-29	- -
30-34	0.1
35-39	1.2
40-44	10.5
45-49	47.2
50-54	146
55-59	321
60-64	553
65-69	835
70-74	894
75-79	806
80-84	609
85+	489

The power law is only rough but it helps to get a handle on what is happening. The simplest explanation of the power (for example about 8 above) is that it relates to the number of mutations needed to produce deadly results; the more mutations needed for a disease, the higher the power. Those with a family history (father, brother) of prostate cancer, have a higher incidence rate because they are born with offending mutations and less time is needed to accrue the necessary number. They are older in a prostate cancer genetic sense than their actual age, and their inherited mutations may have been the more important ones for producing cancer.

A plot of the incidence rate of invasive prostate cancer with age is shown in **Figure 1-2**. There is a low incidence below 50 years of age, with a dramatic increase between the ages of 60 and 70. It peaks in the 70-74 year range, then drops after that but still remains high. A power law behavior does not explain the bending over. The power-law like behavior is the ramping up region up to

Figure 1-2. The incidence rate of *invasive* prostate cancer (2007-2011 data, From the *Seer Cancer Statistics Review 1975-2011*).

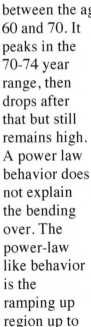
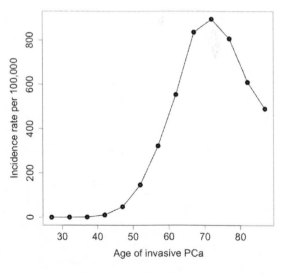

about 70. The important message is that starting in the early

50s, the rate of incidence shoots up reaching a peak around 70-75, and remains high past that but decreases some. The deceleration past 70-75 is very curious, and is not specific to prostate cancer. Decelerations are also seen in many other cancers.

The Trouble-Finding Triad

So how do we find out about Trouble? There is a trouble-finding triad — prostate specific antigen (PSA) screening test, digital rectal exam, and the prostate biopsy. The triad is not perfect, far from it. The PSA test is a blood test usually ordered by your physician as part of a regular (annual) physical exam. The digital rectal exam is also usually performed during your physical exam, and if not, request it. The prostate biopsy is far more involved as it uses a needle to extract specimens of the prostate, which are then analyzed by a pathologist. The needles are administered via the rectum. Are we having fun yet? The prostate biopsy is not part of a regular physical exam, but is called for when there is deep suspicion that the prostate is causing Trouble. All members of the triad can produce false negatives. There are other indicators such as trouble urinating, breaks in urination, blood in urine, and so on. Early diagnosis of Trouble is an important topic, and there are lots of books and literature on the decisions to be made and therapies after diagnosis. Our expedition however is taking us up-river to regions far beyond and more treacherous than these early stages.

There are many experts suggesting that we are over-treating prostate cancer and probably we are. Many prostate cancers are indolent or very slow growing. But the controversy has gone so far as to suggest that PSA screening for healthy men is unnecessary or performed too often. The PSA test is quite imperfect, but let's use what we have and make the best of it. It is a check engine light; maybe you have a problem, maybe it means nothing and is just an annoyance. The situation took a turn for the worse in 2012 when the U.S. Preventive Services Task Force (USPSTF) recommended against prostate specific antigen (PSA) screening for prostate cancer in healthy men. It was given a grade of D, which means it discourages its use. The USPSTF is an independent group of volunteer experts who make recommendations on screenings, counseling, and preventive medications. The argument against screening is that it does not save enough lives, and can cause harm by over-treating the disease. Being crass, it is not a matter of a statistical number of lives, "but will it save yours?" It really comes down to this question: "What is the downside of a PSA test?" And the answer to that is almost nothing, unless the ~$70 cost is your concern. So what is the fuss about? A PSA test is a blood test and can be done at the same time when you are checked for cholesterol, sugars, lipids, liver enzymes and all the rest. The test is data collection, which is far different than treatment.

The real issue is what you do with the information from the PSA test, not the test itself. I'm a believer in taking control, as much as possible, of your own health. You are the stakeholder. You literally live or die with the decisions on what to do. One must educate oneself and seek the best available medical advice on what to do. Sure, the test has false positives indicating there is a problem when there is none. This causes angst for a time. But one can get to the bottom of it fairly quickly. It's better than not checking the engine oil and having the whole engine ("you") seize up.

Informed decision-making is the term used for how decisions are made with the information. You and your physicians (urologist and oncologist) form a team. Your physicians are educated on the matter, but are you? There usually are no black and white decisions, but rather balances between risks and benefits.

Ignorance of prostate cancer is not bliss. I have seen in prostate cancer support groups that men want to be in control of their lives and are vested players in the informed decision-making process. If you decide to get a biopsy performed based on available evidence, and it confirms prostate cancer, a whole new set of decisions arise. At one extreme you can do nothing if you choose, called watchful waiting, or you can swing to the other extreme and have your prostate removed if it is indicated you have a higher-grade cancer. But that decision is your decision, made with the expert opinion of your physician. Whatever is chosen, prostate cancer is now a hot button topic on your watch list, and you will always be on alert for signals suggesting disease progression. No doubt there will be anxiety over this, but if nothing happens to suggest disease progression, go celebrate. Participate in a "Pints for Prostrates" event if so inclined.

PSA is the usual standard used as a biomarker to *monitor progression* once PCa is diagnosed, but it is a more imperfect standard for *diagnosis*. For diagnosis it is of useful utility but not necessarily the best for the job. PSA tests cannot distinguish indolent or aggressive cancer, or tell reliably whether cancer exists at all.

Urologists are usually the first to diagnose, and perhaps treat our Trouble. It is natural then to ask what a urologist would do for diagnosis and initial treatment if he were the patient. A computer-based survey was sent to 2,672 American urologists and there were 215 responses with 198 male. Only 2 did not recommend screening, and only 22 were not sure that screening saves lives. Of the 198 male urologists, 138 had their PSA checked. Those young enough to have never had their PSA checked, 34% plan to have their PSA checked early, between the ages of 40-44. However 11% never plan to have a PSA test. A hypothetical scenario was presented in which they were found to have an elevated PSA and diagnosed with low grade PCa (say Gleason 6). Most (94%) would repeat the PSA test, and about half (48%) would select surveillance.

Light In A Dark Place

Prostate cancer is a dark disease. You may be heading toward a dark place, or are already in a very dark place. You are afraid, scared to death perhaps. We need some light to shine in this dark place and support groups can offer this.

Support groups are unlike anything else you may have experienced. Most members freely discuss their situation, and many have walked in your shoes earlier. You get feedback about what to expect, side effects, coping strategies, and camaraderie with special people—a brotherhood of sorts. Hope can be found. All discussions are to be regarded as confidential. What happens in the support group stays in the support group. There you will be inspired by the courage of others, find that you are not alone, and you will learn about your disease from first-hand accounts. Others may share their experience about a treatment you are about to undertake. UsTOO is the most well known nationally organized group. I am the volunteer facilitator of one group in Arizona.

Prostate cancer disease is not for sissies. It takes courage and resilience. Everyday society tries to hide disease and illness. Being with others in your situation reminds us that we are not alone. We learn to stop—there are roses to smell, birds to admire, trees to marvel at and stars to remind us of our small place in an unlimited universe. A special gift comes with each day. Never let anyone ruin your day. It's your day, your gift, and you own it, not someone else. Someone that cuts you off in traffic is too busy to smell the roses, as their universe is stuck only within themselves. Don't let them or anyone else upset you or take-away even a minute of your precious day.

It is hard to understand why prostate cancer has decided to pay you a visit. It can turn into the "Why me?" syndrome. Did you do something wrong? It can happen to anyone. Chemist Linus Pauling 1901-1994, a winner of two Nobel prizes (Chemistry and Peace), both unshared, and arguably one of the greatest chemists of the 20th century, died of prostate cancer. He died of a ripe old age, so he did a fairly good job of outrunning it. He followed the Credo. But it can happen to anyone.

Prostate Cancer And Breast Cancer

Prostate cancer in men and breast cancer in women have many common aspects. Both organs require gonadal steroids to function and develop— either estrogen or androgen. These hormones exist in both men and women, but are expressed at different levels in the two sexes. Breast cancer tumors are driven by estrogen, while prostate cancer tumors are driven by androgen (e.g. testosterone). Both cancers have receptors that are activated by hormones. The estrogen receptors are ERα and ERβ, while for prostate cells it is the androgen receptor (AR). We will detail the AR later, as it is a major player in prostate cancer. For now we only need to realize that these receptors head to the cancer cell nucleus to activate its DNA, causing expression of genes for cell growth and replication. Since these two cancers are, at least in early progression, hormone sensitive, they have treatments that have similarities—hormone therapies. Additionally both cancers, if they metastasize, preferentially target lymph nodes and bone. A benefit of the similarities of these two cancers is that research and breakthroughs in one cancer can sometimes benefit the other. But it is not so simple.

Prostate cancer in men is more prevalent than breast cancer in women. Each year 218,000 men are diagnosed with prostate cancer and 209,000 women are diagnosed with breast cancer. But women are more likely to die yearly from breast cancer than men are from prostate cancer—40,000 women die from breast cancer while 32,000 men from prostate cancer. The mortality numbers are different but not wildly different. However, buzz about breast cancer appears to be an order of magnitude larger than for prostate cancer.

Unfortunately, "buzz" imbalance is also evident in the National Institutes of Health (NIH) government funding. This agency is "the" agency responsible for scientific funding of disease cause and cure. Funding levels from the NIH in FY2013 were $286M for PCa and $657M for breast cancer—quite an imbalance for fairly similar mortality and diagnosis rates. Part of the bias is that prostate cancer is an "old man's disease," while breast cancer has an equal opportunity component. These biases are evident in a CSPAN interview by Brian Lamb of Dr. Francis Collins, Director of the National Institutes of Health, on March 2013. Here Dr. Collins referred to differences in public health emergencies of the two diseases. Women's advocacy has made breast cancer a public health emergency.

On the positive side, men owe a debt to women's activism. Prostate cancer may have been even more ignored if it were not for women's successful advocacy. Prostate cancer is slowly being noticed, and the situation has improved even since 2013. There are now many active groups (e.g. UsTOO, Malecare, ZeroCancer, and National Alliance of State Prostate Cancer Coalitions). The prostate cancer sky blue ribbon now complements the familiar pink ribbon for breast cancer.

Off We Go On The Journey To Explore Trouble

Please step on the keelboat for our expedition with care; the going will be rough at times. We will first gather more provisions, which for advanced prostate cancer is the science concerning hormone therapy. Then we leave our home base travelling on keelboat upstream and explore the waters of some new therapies the FDA has approved in the last 5-10 years. These waters show the role of the androgen receptor, which lead to the new drugs Enzalutamide and Abiraterone Acetate. Our waters will be infested with the science behind these advances. This produces a coveted map of prostate cancer's underbelly that is necessary for future expeditions. The science will at times seem like paddling upstream. We will reach the end of the water, leaving our keelboats behind and must explore the rocky terrain of developing therapies, including immunotherapy. Perhaps one of these will lead to a cure or near cure, or perhaps not. Like Lewis and Clark, we will attempt to survive the tough winter

20

of our disease, make it over the Rockies and find a downstream flow to the Pacific.

And please remember that the material covered is for informational purposes only. Always (always!) consult a medical professional for what treatments, therapies, and medications are best for you.

References

Imaging in Oncology from The University of Texas M. D. Anderson Cancer Center: Diagnosis, Staging, and Surveillance of Prostate Cancer, V Kundra, PM Silverman, SF Matin and H Choi, American Journal of Roentgenology 189(4), 830-844 (2007).

High prevalence of prostatic neoplasia in Australian men, MM Orde, NJ Whitaker and JS Lawson, Pathology, 41(5), 433-5 (2009).

Cancer statistics, CA , A. Jemal, R. Siegel, J. Xu and E. Ward, A Cancer Journal for Clinicians 60, 277–300 (2010).

Deaths: Leading Causes for 2010, M. Heron, National Vital Statistics Reports 62(6), 1-96 (2013).

An estimation of the number of cells in the human body, E Bianconi et al., Annals of Human Biology 40(6), 463-471 (2013).

Copy number analysis indicates monoclonal origin of lethal metastatic prostate cancer, W Liu et al., Nature Medicine 15(5), 559-565 (2009).

Analytical validation of the Oncotype DX prostate cancer assay – a clinical RT-PCR assay optimized for prostate needle biopsies, D Knezevic, et al., BMC Genomics 2013, 14, 690-701 (2013).

Age incidence curves for cancer (somatic utation/epigenetic changes), GS Watson, Proceedings of the National Academy of Science USA, 74(4), 1341-1342 (1977).

Age Distribution of Cancer: The Incidence Turnover at Old Age, F Pompei and R Wilson, Human and Ecological Risk Assessment 7(6), 1619-1650 (2001).

Urologists' personal feelings on PSA screening and prostate cancer treatment, DL Wenzler and BH Rosenberg, Journal of Evaluation in Clinical Practice, 20(4), 408-410 (2014).

Chapter 2

Standard Care Of Trouble

A woman brought her child with an abscess in the lower part of the back, and offered as much corn as she could carry for some medicine; we administered to it of course very cheerfully. Meriwether Lewis, 1804.

There are standard treatments of advanced or metastatic prostate cancer. The medical community incorporates changes each year to update physicians to advancements that are made. Changes not only include new therapies, but also the timing or sequencing of therapies. This information comes from clinical trials that are in progress or completed and that have been proven to work, at least to a certain extent.

Cancer is an individualist disease and each person has their own characteristic version, so you and your physician may decide on significant modifications from the "vanilla-flavor" standard of care. For example, the European Urological Association (EAU) has a set of guidelines that they recommend physicians adhere to, but compliance is far from uniform with only a 30-40% compliance rate.

The first weapon that is applied to almost all advanced prostate cancers is androgen ablation, also known as androgen deprivation therapy (ADT). This therapy is usually effective but is only so for a while. The disease usually progresses to a hormone refractory form (better described as hormone resistant or castrate resistant), with a mean time in the general ballpark of 36 months. The origin of this resistance is clear (Chapter 3). Keep in mind that mean times are only statistical; different cohorts of patients yield different statistics and know that statistics are just that, statistics. You are not a statistic. There are individual factors that greatly affect progression time to castrate resistance. Some take many years, some take only one year. When cancer progresses to castrate resistant prostate cancer (CRPC), or its metastatic version (mCRPC), the cancer no longer responds to standard androgen deprivation. One attempts to take away the cancer's "car keys," yet it still progresses. As we will see later, CRPC still is in fact dependent on androgens (usually) but ADT is not enough to control it.

The seriousness of PCa is ratcheted up to the next level when it becomes castrate resistant. There have been several new treatments for CRPC that have undergone large-scale clinical trials that are proven to be partially effective in extending overall survival. I say partially effective because prostate cancer warriors still find it despairing. There is a long way to go before we can find rest. The advances have overall percentage survival increases of 20-50%, but still median overall survival in several trials is just 2 or 3 or 4 years. New treatments of CRPC and mCRPC that have occurred in the last few years give us hope by scratching the surface (but just barely) of a cure. Each small increase in understanding can lead to a much-improved therapy and the prospect of a much improved and enduring remission.

Table 2-1 shows the main weapons used in the treatment of advanced prostate cancer. There are many other therapies that we will discuss—the table shows the heavy hitters. One notices that there have been several new additions since 2010. This increase in new therapies is an encouraging sign for the future. The hope is that we get to a better future before it is too late for many of us, and we can satisfy the PCa credo of dying from something else.

The Standard – Androgen Deprivation Therapy (ADT)

Standard treatment of androgen responsive PCa is androgen ablation, that is the removal of androgen (mainly testosterone and dihydrotestosterone). This can be done medically by castration, but in the U.S. this is usually done chemically. Whew—we dodged that bullet! Chemically it is called Gonadotropin Releasing Hormone (GnRH) or by the

Table 2-1	Treatment	Action/Purpose	FDA approval/Chapter
Androgen deprivation therapy, ADT. Leuprolide (Lupron), Degarelix (Firmagon)		Leuprolide/Degarelix inhibits the production of testosterone.	1986 Luteinizing hormone-releasing hormone (LHRH) androgen deprivation therapy. Chapter 2
Enzalutamide (Xtandi)		Antiandrogen: inhibits androgen activation of the androgen receptor.	2012 Metastatic castrate resistant PCa after docetaxel. 2014 Metastatic castrate resistant PCa before docetaxel. Chapter 4.
Abiraterone acetate (Zytiga) + prednisone.		Block androgen synthesis.	2011, Chapter 5.
Sipuleucel-T (Provenge)		Immunotherapy	2010, Chapter 13.
Radium 223 (Xofigo)		Internal radiation of bone metastases.	2013, Chapter 8.
Denosumab (Xgeva). Also bisphosphonates.		To help prevent bone damage from bone metastases and ADT	2010, Chapter 8.
Docetaxel (Taxotere)		1st line Chemotherapy that inhibits cell reproduction.	2004, Chapter 9.
Cabazitaxel (Jevtana)		2nd line Chemotherapy that inhibits cell reproduction.	2010, Chapter 9.
Cisplatin		A powerful chemo drug for very aggressive cancer.	----, Chapter 9.

older name Luteinizing Hormone-Releasing Hormone (LHRH) androgen deprivation therapy. (I will be using both names – GnRH for newer work and LHRH for the historical developments that led to two Nobel Prizes.) This is quite effective for hormone responding cancers; before prostate cancer becomes castrate resistant (CRPC). Androgen deprivation therapy (ADT) is usually the first significant therapy used.

ADT is tried and true. Unfortunately it does not cure, but is a delay strategy. Charles Huggins uncovered the scientific underpinnings in 1941 while studying prostate cancer. This was at a time before the PSA biomarker. The blood serum biomarker of that day was the enzyme prostatic acid phosphatase (PAP), the same protein that is used today to target cancer prostate cancer cells with the immunotherapy Sipuleucel-T (Provenge). Alexander and Ethel Gutman discovered PAP just a few years earlier in the late 1930s. They found that prostate cancer sufferers had high levels of this enzyme in their blood serum. Prostate cancer research was on a roll just before WWII broke out.

Huggins was studying metastatic prostate cancer and found that "decreasing the activity of androgens through castration or estrogenic injections" produced a reduction in PAP serum levels. Today we monitor religiously our PSA levels instead to see if the disease is progressing or relapsing. Huggins also purposely increased androgen levels and found increased PAP levels in blood. This was the first observation that hormones and prostate cancer growth were correlated. The paper was entitled "Studies on prostatic cancer, I. The effect of castration, estrogen and androgen injection on serum phosphatases in metastatic carcinoma of the prostate."

We think we are so smart today with all our highly engineered biotechnology equipment and concepts. But this discovery made over 70 years ago is still the first line of defense we have today against prostate cancer. Huggins believed "It is the genius of research to frame a question so simply that a conditional answer is prohibited." Many of today's prostate cancer drugs have overall survival increases of months—hormone therapy often has overall survival increases of many years. Let's not lose sight of the fact that sometimes the most important developments, in hindsight, often seem simple.

Charles Huggins and team member/former student Clarence Hodges are true pioneers in our Lewis and Clark-like expedition. Charles Huggins received the Nobel Prize in Physiology/Medicine in 1966 *"for his discoveries concerning hormonal treatment of prostatic cancer."* The Prize was shared with another cancer giant, Peyton Rous *"for his discovery of tumor-inducing viruses."* Charles Huggins died in 1997 at the ripe old age of 95.

At the 1966 Nobel Prize Ceremony, it was mentioned that Rous understood the significance of Huggins' work and wrote *"the importance of this discovery* (androgen deprivation) *far transcends its practical implications; for it means that thought and endeavor in cancer research have been misdirected in consequence of the belief that tumor cells are anarchic."* This comment helps take us back to the thinking back in 1941 about cancer in general, that cancer followed no rules but anarchy. Prostate cancer does follow rules, rules that healthy prostate cells may not follow. It is our job to find what rulebook they use and use these rules to end their game.

What androgen deprivation therapy is all about is reducing androgens, mainly testosterone. The route to do this is somewhat circuitous (See **Figure 2-1**). The hypothalamus in the brain is a link between the central nervous system and hormones. It releases regulating hormones that cause other hormones to be produced or to stop being produced. One of these regulating hormones is Gonadotropin Releasing Hormone (GnRH also known as LHRH). This hormone is taken up by receptors in the pituitary gland and signals the pituitary to produce Luteinizing Hormone (LH). LH signals the testes to produce testosterone, the main androgen we are wishing to remove in androgen deprivation therapy. The testes produce about 95% of the testosterone, and 5% of the androgens are produced by the adrenal. The androgens are taken up by the androgen receptors that exist within prostate cells in the prostate or prostate cancer lesions and get the cells fired up.

Other actors in the figure are ACTH and Prolactin. Adrenocorticotropic hormone (ACTH) triggers the adrenal

Figure 2-1. Pathways leading to the production of testosterone and androgens. More details in J-E Damber, Acta Oncologica 44, 605-609 (2005).

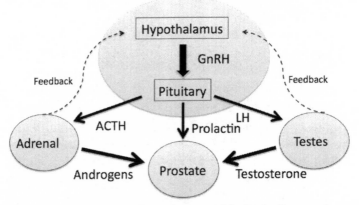

gland to produce adrenal corticosteroids including androgens like the powerful androgen dihydrotestosterone (DHT). Prolactin has many functions (for example lactation in women), including being a growth factor for the prostate and also influences the androgen receptor.

A big step was accomplished in determining that the hypothalamus and pituitary were at the core of the control system. Knowing how it works is not only cerebrally satisfying, but knowledge is power. This knowledge offers targets to interrupt the control system to reduce testosterone synthesis. This brings us to the second half of our story. The heroes of this part of the story are Andrew V. Schally and Roger Guillemin who shared one half of the Nobel Prize in Physiology or Medicine in 1977 "for their discoveries concerning the peptide hormone production of the brain."

The Nobel Prize was awarded quickly after their work. In 1971 they discovered that Luteinizing Hormone-

Releasing Hormone (LHRH, GnRH) from the hypothalamus regulates the Luteinizing Hormone from the pituitary. It was also found that LHRH simultaneously regulates the follicle-stimulating hormone (FSH). Just two year later in 1973 the structure of the LHRH amino-acid peptide was unraveled. This led the way to synthetic versions, called LHRH analogues, with improved properties that are used today.

FDA approval of LHRH in advanced PCa occurred in 1986, nine years after the Nobel Prize. This episode appears to have occurred quickly by medical standards, but to be just, Schally began working in this area in the 1950s. He submitted his Ph.D. thesis "In *vitro* studies on the control of the release of ACTH" in 1957. So his trailblazing began much earlier.

It helps to know what the words luteinizing hormone-releasing hormone (LHRH) mean to help our understanding of their mechanism of action. The word Lutein is Latin for luteus, which means yellow. In this context it is referring to the yellow color of a family of carotenoid biochemicals that gives carrots their color and (partly) their health benefits. The process of luteinizing originally referred to the production of the corpus luteum (yellow body) in women during each menstrual cycle related to progesterone and estrogen hormone production. The term then carries over to men. A luteinizing hormone is one that affects the production of sexual hormones. The key concept is that men release luteinizing hormone from the pituitary and that signals the testes to produce testosterone.

It came as a bonus to PCa sufferers that LHRH was found to induce mating in rats. This immediately brought to mind that LHRH might help men with infertility. Sex sells and this produced an added incentive for others to get in the LHRH game and advance the field for PCa.

Unraveling the action of LHRH and its chemical composition was no simple project. Schally in his Noble lecture, tells us about the difficulty in obtaining pure LHRH to study it: "The first isolation of 800 μg (0.8 mg) LHRH/FSHRH from ventral hypothalami of *165,000* pigs was achieved by twelve successive purification steps which included ..." (emphasis mine). That's a lot of pig hypothalami. But one need to the pure material to determine what it is and to synthesize it in the laboratory so that pigs are no longer needed. We have pigs to thank for ADT.

So what did Schally find LHRH (GnRH) to be? We will discuss proteins in more detail in Chapter 6, but we need to know a little at this stage. Proteins are a string of amino acids forming one long molecule. Amino acids are small molecules that can be stacked together with common molecular glue called a peptide bond. There are 20 naturally occurring amino acids and exactly the way they are ordered gives the protein its uniqueness, just like the 26 letters of the alphabet give words and sentences. Proteins make amazing machines, and "machines" is appropriate. But LHRH is not quite a protein. It contains just 10 amino acids, and when they are that small they are called peptides, or polypeptides, for they are not big enough to form machines like enzymes. But peptides can convey a signal by binding to a receptor — and in this case they signal the pituitary. Mother Nature's LHRH is a deca-peptide (10) of composition:
Human LHRH

pGlu-His-Trp-Ser-Tyr-Gly-Leu-Arg-Pro-GlyNH$_2$
1   2   3   4   5   6   7   8   9   10

which is a standard shorthand for Glutamic Acid (1), Histidine (2), Tryptophan (3), Serine (4), Tyrosine (5), Glycine (6), Leucine (7), Arginine (8), Proline (9), Glycine (10). The ends of the deca-peptide are slightly non-standard. pGlu is a slight variation of Glutamic acid (Pyroglutamic acid) and GlyNH2 is an amide (nitrogen containing) end terminated Gly. (Don't sweat details. It's just a soup of letters for a complex chemical.)

The most common synthetic analogue of human LHRH in use today is Leuprolide Acetate (Lupron). Its structure is:
Leuprolide

pGlu-His-Trp-Ser-Tyr-**DLeu**-Leu-Arg-Pro-**NHEt**
1   2   3   4   5   6   7   8   9   10

where NHEt is the chemical N-ethylamide. There are two amino acid changes from that of Mother Nature—one at position 6 and the other at position 10. One might ask "Why try to improve on Mother Nature by making changes?" The answer is that Mother Nature is not attempting to deal with prostate cancer, but we are. Natural LHRH has a half-life in the blood of only 3-4 minutes. The hypothalamus pulses out LHRH in bursts and it is to act on the pituitary quickly. Digestive enzymes break up Mother Nature's peptide chain, primarily at positions 6 and position 10. The changes allow for protection from these breaks and for greater binding in the LHRH receptors in the pituitary.

One notes that D-Leucine (D for dextro, right-handed) in position 6 of the Leuprolide is a right-handed amino acid. Left-handed and right-handed molecules are mirror images of each other. Amino acids made by the human body are left-handed, and our bodily processing of amino acids is designed for left-handed varieties. So sneaking in a right-handed molecule causes a reduced effectiveness of the enzymes that break it up.

Possible Strategies

Figure 2-1 shows that testosterone is released from the testes and the adrenal glands. There are many ways that this information can be used to stop the production of androgen to stop fueling the prostate cancer in the prostate or metastatic sites.

The most obvious step is to surgically remove the testes, an orchidectomy. This is one of the options that Huggins had available in 1941. It works, but men, especially younger men, are very reluctant to have this done—for good reason in my estimation. Our testes have served us well, and represent more than testosterone factories. They possibly produced children that maybe led to grandchildren. That is no way to treat a trusted friend.

A friendlier target is downstream of the testes and that is to change how testosterone (androgens) influences the prostate or prostate cancer cells. This is where many of the newer therapies are working and is where much of current research occurs. These will be covered later on when we explore the androgen receptor.

A strategy upstream of the testes is to influence the hypothalamus to stop producing GnRH. That is done by the administration of estrogen. This option was also available to Huggins in 1941, and is still used today. It causes the hypothalamus to reduce the secretion of GnRH. This prevents ultimate signaling of the testes, and is a viable strategy except that estrogen, the female hormone, causes some undesirable side effects that limit its use.

Also upstream from the testes is the pituitary that secretes LH and FSH. The pituitary is a great target to stop the production of androgen, and is the principal component of androgen depravation therapy. We certainly do not directly interfere with the pituitary (or the hypothalamus for that matter) since they control so many endocrine functions. We could cause all types of unintended consequences doing that. But we can use the fact that the hypothalamus signals the pituitary without caustically interfering with them.

Both agonist and antagonists of pituitary receptors, GnRH (LHRH) receptors, accomplish this. Hold on — **agonists activate, and antagonists inhibit**. So which one works? It's curious and confusing that these two strategies are, at first blush, completely opposite strategies and they both work. Inhibiting the receptor with an antagonist stops stimulation of the pituitary; this causes it to stop secreting LH so the testes are not stimulated. But an agonist stimulates the receptor to produce LH, thus stimulating the testes to produce androgen. Agonists are used routinely for ADT therapy, while antagonists are becoming serious competitors. Let's now look at both of these strategies.

The Agonist Strategy

The answer to the agonist versus antagonist paradox is that the agonists, which stimulate the pituitary, stimulate it so much that it saturates the pituitary's receptors. This causes a spike in LH and FSH secretion, but then it drops off in a few days. Our system is designed to receive brief pulses of GnRH on a scale of 1.5-2.0 hours apart. But we administer

GnRH agonists for PCa quite differently. We supply a constant supply of GnRH due to the increased lifetime of the synthetic peptide, its increased concentration, and packaging that allows it to be time released. This produces quite a different response. There is a spike in LH secretion that produces an initial spike in testosterone. This is undesirable but is usually made less important by taking an antiandrogen (like bicalutamide (Casodex), nilutamide, or glutamide) to block the androgen receptor from the testosterone spike and prevent stimulation of prostate cancer cells. Antiandrogens are usually started before the GnRH agonist is administered.

The GnRH agonists used for ADT are Leuprolide Acetate (Lupron, Eligard), Buserelin (Suprefact) and Goserelin (Zoladex). This form of ADT treatment has been the most popular treatment for advanced PCa for nearly 30 years. The first GnHR agonist to be approved was in 1986. The goal is to get testosterone levels in blood serum to castration levels, which is less than around 0.2ng/mL (nanogram per milliliter). Another unit sometimes used is ng/dL (nanogram per deciliter). A dL is 100mL. Thus 0.2ng/mL is equivalent to 20ng/dL.

The androgen receptor (Chapter 3) is the biologic protein in prostate cells that uptakes androgen and promotes cell growth. The name of the game in ADT is to stop androgen from ever getting to the androgen receptor. Besides attempting to stop androgen production, we can also block what remaining androgen is produced from joining with the receptor. These are antiandrogens (or androgen blockers). Antiandrogens like bicalutamide (Casodex) are used with GnRH antagonists to form a double blockade.

One can go further and produce a triple blockade by adding a third drug that is a 5-alpha reductase inhibitor. More on 5-alpha reductase will be given in Chapter 5. These drugs, such as Dutasteride (Avodart) or Proscar (Finasteride), inhibit the formation of dihydrotestosterone from testosterone. Dihydrotestosterone (DHT) is an especially bad actor in that it is far more potent in activating the androgen receptor. Chemically this means it has a higher binding affinity with the receptor. Activation of the androgen receptor ultimately promotes prostate cancer cell growth. [FYI: Androgen receptors are a key to prostate cancer and they are covered in Chapter 3. The biosynthesis of the androgen steroids and the role of 5-alpha reductase will be covered in Chapter 5.]

Generally prostate cancer grows and divides being promoted by androgens such as testosterone, as androgens activate the androgen receptor within the prostate cell. Upon activation it causes the cell to grow and reproduce. Removing testosterone stunts the disease progression, at least for a while. This treatment is usually very effective and if prostate cancer would not alter itself to be resistant to androgen or independent of external androgen, all would be fine. But prostate cancer presents itself as a moving target. What we hope for is at least a slowly moving target.

Some men have real trouble with the side effects of ADT. It is no picnic, but compared to the alternative, perhaps it is actually a box lunch. Side effects include weight gain, enlarged breasts, hot flashes, loss of sexual desire and function, mental fog, and fatigue. It's hard to accept going from Mr. Stud to Mr. Dud. I did not experience mental fog too significantly, perhaps because I lived my whole life in one. I for one vote for fatigue and weight gain as the most undesirable. Additionally there is a certain feeling of being turned into a woman. Those who have a radical prostatectomy (removal of the prostate) also have one of their urinary sphincters removed. This makes the feeling even more complete as women only have one urinary sphincter to begin with. One sphincter makes us more prone to leakage. These are more inconveniences and discomforts rather than serious side effects.

Some may be appalled that I downplay the side effects of ADT. We are talking about a serious disease with death possibly being a not too distant "side effect." In contrast, loss of sexual function doesn't sound so bad after all. With ADT you also lose much of the desire, a curious form of good news considering your sexual performance is seriously compromised. Put crassly, the bad news is you can't, the good news is you don't want to.

But there are potential very serious side effects. Androgens help build muscle and bone mass. Loss of bone mass is of course dangerous, producing osteopenia and osteoporosis. This can lead to bone fractures including of the hip. Additionally, there is the double whammy for those suffering from metastatic PCa in the bone of an additional risk of fractures due to compromises of bone due to bone lesions. Then there is the issue of ADT promoting heart disease. Stop! This book is not about side effects, as its content would balloon uncontrollably if so. This type of information is easy to find and there are plenty of books on the topic. Each patient must do his own due diligence on this topic.

The Antagonist Strategy

Both GnRH agonists and antagonists are used to stop the release of luteinizing hormone, which in turn drastically turns down the production of testosterone in the testes. Although these two statements appear contradictory, both are true. They act in different ways and **Figure 2-2** clearly shows the difference in operation. Agonists (like Leuprolide) **stimulate** the pituitary to initially produce luteinizing hormone (LH) and follicle stimulating hormone (FSH), but overstimulation of the pituitary causes it to shut down this production after 1-3 weeks. Antagonists (like Degarelix) on the other hand **block** the LHRH receptor, so that it cannot be stimulated in the first place. This is a direct stoppage of LH and FSH production.

The advantages of an **antagonist** are clear. Blockers produce a near immediate cessation of LH production, which then causes the testes to stop producing testosterone. **Agonists** act more slowly and the testosterone reduction may take 2-3 weeks to be accomplished. This will be reflected in PSA levels. Additionally, in some cases, spikes in LH and thus testosterone may occur upon repeated treatments with agonists, but not an antagonist. Temporary testosterone flare-ups and PSA rises certainly do not seem beneficial.

34

GnRH **antagonist** has a natural appeal and gives a more favorable testosterone and PSA response. There are other advantages of LHRH antagonists (blockers) as well.

So why are **agonists** used more often than **antagonists** when antagonists seem to have advantages? It appears there are four reasons, but the reasons are rapidly

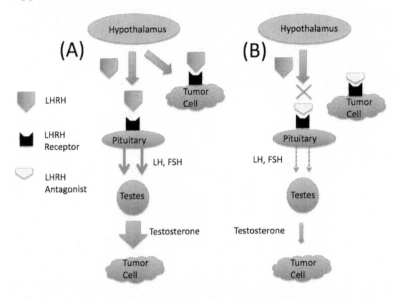

Figure 2-2. How an LHRH antagonist works. (A) The normal signaling process. The hypothalamus releases LHRH, which is received by receptors in the pituitary that ultimately cause production of testosterone. 86% of prostate cancer cells express the LHRH receptor, which are also activated by LHRH. (B) An LHRH antagonist blocks the LHRH receptor in the pituitary reducing the production of testosterone, and cells expressing the LHRH receptor. More details in FG Rick et al., Oncology Targets and Therapy 6, 391–402 (2013).

being displaced. The reasons are: slow start, reduced track history, inertia, and less convenient delivery.

The first and most powerful reason is that antagonists got off to a slow, and perhaps wrong, start. The first LHRH blocker Abarelix (Plenaxis) was approved in

2003, but it was found that in some men it might have caused a release of histamine. This can produce anaphylaxis allergic reaction. Swelling, itching, and serious breathing impairments can result. Marketing was stopped in the U.S.A. in 2005, although it is still possible to get it outside the U.S. Those that started on Abarelix can still get it in the U.S.; a sensible decision since anaphylaxis has not been a problem with them, so far.

So it was back to the drawing board for LHRH blockers. The FDA approved the third-generation blocker FE200486, now called Degarelix Acetate (Firmagon) in 2008. This drug reduced considerably the histamine production. But 2008 is not so long ago compared to the agonist leuprolide acetate that obtained its first U.S.A. approval for monthly injections in 1989. That's the reduced track record reason. Leuprolide has a long history, while Degarelix does not. This means that the long-term results are still not in. This makes physicians, and more importantly patients, nervous.

The third reason is simply inertia—Newton's first law of motion applied to medicine. If the agonist Leuprolide is working, current patients are reluctant to change unless there are substantial benefits. Physicians, too, may not want to chance what has been working for them with something they are less familiar with. Every choice one makes along this journey has pros and cons. New patients will probably be more inclined to try a blocker. The short-term results and some near term results are in and they appear favorable for Degarelix.

The fourth and final reason that there is hesitation in using Degarelix compared to Leuprolide is convenience in administration. Degarelix is administered as a deep subcutaneous injection in the abdominal region, which can be painful if not done properly. Sometimes there are reactions at the injection site. Degarelix is administered every 28 days, which means frequent doctor's office visits. In contrast Leuprolide is administered as an intramuscular injection (e.g. a shot in the buttocks) that has almost no sensation. Leuprolide has various dosages, and application schedules vary. It can be several months between injections; this reduces physician office visits.

There are significant differences in follicle stimulating hormone (FSH) release between the agonist and the antagonist approach. FSH release is stopped in both approaches, but with an agonist there is sometimes FSH escape, where FSH gradually begins to rise. In the 1990s agonists were being considered as a male contraceptive, but FSH escape would still cause the production of sperm. That's a huge problem for that application. The whole idea of ADT for contraception appears desperate, as ADT is a serious change in male hormone balance. It is one that is justifiable for advanced PCa, which is a life-threatening situation. But contraception—are there not reasonable alternatives?

The advantage of FSH reduction for PCa is not fully understood. Prostate cancer cells do take FSH in and this could promote tumor growth. Receptors for FSH are more frequently expressed on cancerous prostate cells than healthy prostate cells. It has been suggested that FSH plays a role in the regulation of growth of castrate-resistant prostate cancer. FSH also may play a role in accelerating bone loss, a problem already occurring from lack of testosterone, ADT, and metastatic lesions. (See the review by Shore et al. for more details on FSH.) These indications appear to come down on the side of completely removing FSH, which is accomplished well by a blocker such as Degarelix.

A phase III clinical trial (CS21) was performed on Degarelix for treatment for advanced prostate cancer. The primary outcome was to reduce testosterone levels in the blood to castration levels over a 12-month period. Castration level in this study is defined as less than 50ng/dL (equivalent to 0.5ng/mL). There were three groups—two taking the antagonist Degarelix and the third taking the agonist Leuprolide (with 11% also taking Bicalutamide). Castration levels were kept at a 98.3-97.2% for those in the blocker Degarelix groups with the range depending on Degarelix dose. The Leuprolide cohort had a castration-level success rate after one year of 96.4%. Although the 1-2% advantage is a benefit, the real point is that both methods are fairly effective. In the medical literature they would say Degarelix (the competitor to the established treatment) was not inferior to Leuprolide. There were more reactions at the injection site, which occurred in roughly one-third of the Degarelix patients, and almost none of the Leuprolide patients.

The project was extended past the one-year mark and is continuing. There are no results yet for overall survival differences (the long-term problem), but there are results for progression free survival (PFS), defined here as either the lack of PSA progression or death, obviously one being far worse than the other. There was a difference between those

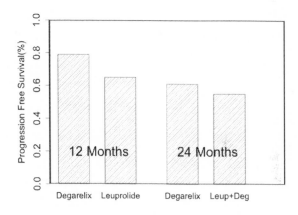

Figure 2-3. Results of the CS21 trial showing the probability of progression free survival (PFS) after 12 months upon taking either Degarelix or Leuprolide as first line ADT. Degarelix showed an advantage after one year. After 1 year, those on Leuprolide changed to Degarelix. The two groups are becoming more equal in PFS after 24 months. After B Tombal et al., European Urology 57, 836-842 (2010).

patients with a starting PSA greater than 20ng/ml (higher risk) and those with lower PSA levels before ADT treatment. The extension had the interesting twist that after one year, patients could switch from Leuprolide to the blocker Degarelix. **Figure 2-3** shows the probability of progression free survival for the high-risk subset (>20ng/ml initial PSA). All patients shown in the bar graph are taking Degarelix after 12 months.

The results are quite remarkable in several ways. First note that after one year the Progression Free Survival probability (lack of PSA failure or death) of 70-80% is far less favorable than the 96%+ rate of castration levels of testosterone (obviously from those that did not die). But on the positive side, the Degarelix cohort did better than the Leuprolide group the first year. But most remarkable of all, when changing from Leuprolide, the agonist, to the (antagonist) blocker Degarelix, the two groups begin to achieve similar progression-free survival rates. Thus if you make it to a year on an agonist, it's not too late to change to an antagonist. That is if you dare—you made it that far without progression, and inertia is hard to overcome.

References

EAU guidelines on prostate cancer. Part II: treatment of advanced, relapsing, and castrate resistance prostate cancer, A Heidenreich, et al., European Urology 65, 467-479 (2014). (www.uroweb.org)

Studies on prostatic cancer, I. The effect of castration, estrogen and androgen injection on serum phosphatases in metastatic carcinoma of the prostate, C Huggins and CV Hodges, Cancer Research 1, 293-297 (1941).

Studies on prostatic cancer: II. The effects of castration on advanced carcinoma of the prostate gland, C Huggins, RE Stevens Jr and CV Hodges, Archives of Surgery 43, 209-223 (1941).

Endocrine therapy for prostate cancer, J-E Damber, Acta Oncologica 44, 605-609 (2005).

Reassessment of the definition of castrate levels of testosterone: implications for clinical decision making, MG Oefelein, A Feng, MJ Scolieri, D Ricchiutti, MI Resnick, Urology 56, 1021-1024 (2000).

Follicle-Stimulating Hormone (FSH) Escape During Chronic Gonadotropin-Releasing Hormone (GnRH) Agonist and Testosterone Treatment, S Bhasin, N Berman and RS Swerdloff, Journal of Andrology 15 (5), 386-391 (1994).

An update on the use of degarelix in the treatment of advanced hormone-dependent prostate cancer, FG Rick, NL Block, and Andrew V Schally, Oncology Targets and Therapy 6, 391–402 (2013).

REVIEW: New considerations for ADT in advanced prostate cancer and the emerging role of GnRH antagonists, ND Shore, P-A Abrahamsson, J Anderson, ED Crawford and P Lange, Prostate Cancer and Prostatic Diseases 16, 7-15 (2013).

Optimal Control of Testosterone: A Clinical Case-Based Approach of Modern Androgen-Deprivation Therapy, B Tombal and R Berges, European Urology Supplements 7, 15–21 (2008).

A phase III extension trial with a one-arm crossover from leuprolide to degarelix: comparison of gonadotropin-releasing hormone agonist and antagonist effect on prostate cancer, ED Crawford, B Tombal, K Miller, L Boccon-Gibod, F Schroder, N Shore et al., Journal of Urology 186, 889–897 (2011).

Additional analysis of the secondary end point of biochemical recurrence rate in a phase 3 trial (CS21) comparing degarelix 80mg versus leuprolide in prostate cancer patients segmented by baseline characteristics, B Tombal, K Miller, L Boccon-Gibod, F Schroder, N Shore, ED Crawford et al., European Urology 57, 836-842 (2010).

The efficacy and safety of degarelix: a 12-month, comparative, randomized, openlabel, parallel-group phase III study in patients with prostate cancer L Klotz, L Boccon-Gibod, ND Shore, C Andreou, BE Persson, P. Cantor P et al., British Journal of Urology International 102, 1531-1538 (2008).

Chapter 3

Big Trouble Caused By The Androgen Receptor (AR)

If you know the problem, that's half the battle to coming up with the solution. That's the source of creativity. Eric Betzig, 2014 Nobel Prize in Chemistry

Androgen hormone deprivation therapy is usually effective in stalling the progression of metastatic prostate cancer. The cancer cells are hormone sensitive and the removal of androgen causes them to retreat. After a year or two or three or ..., androgen deprivation is no longer effective and PCa progresses. The cancer cells are "hormone insensitive," and the disease is called hormone refractory, hormone resistant, or castrate resistant PCa (CRPC). It was thought that the cancer cells no longer needed testosterone or DHT to grow and multiply. Marvelous work in 2004 from University of California Los Angeles showed that this is not the case. They also showed several other surprises — surprises that when understood led to the discovery of new treatments and drugs such as the 2013 FDA approval of Enzalutamide. The hero of this chapter and the leader of the 2004 UCLA work is Charles L. Sawyers.

It is this work and the surprises that we explore in this chapter. A protein called the androgen receptor rules the dense brush that we will be hacking our way through along our expedition. The androgen receptor, or AR for short, is a 919 amino acid protein. Its important job is to regulate gene expression, particularly those "manly" genes regulated by male sex hormones.

It sounds harmless enough, but the androgen receptor (AR) allows androgens like testosterone or DHT to activate prostate cancer cells. Before the cell went cancerous, the AR had a normal function in androgen-activated processes. But once the cell becomes cancerous, we would like the AR to turn off. If we can learn how to control the AR, then maybe we have a chance of controlling the cancer.

Androgen receptors are surprising in the way they act—very surprising. A clear understanding of the AR leads to a better understanding of ways to control prostate cancer. But getting this information has been a long scientific haul. Backtracking this haul will be our task in this chapter.

It was thought that the refractory cancer cells no longer needed testosterone or DHT to grow and multiply. Previous to the work described in this chapter, this is what was believed to cause refractory behavior. Three possibilities: 1) Mutations in the AR gene. Most patients (at least early on in CRPC) do not have AR mutations. 2) Increased kinase signaling mediated by oncogenes causes the AR to be activated without an androgen. 3) New pathways have opened up and the AR is no longer part of the growth and survival of the cell. The critical point is that there was considerable debate over what causes androgen refractory behavior (CRPC).

The important job of the AR is to regulate **gene expression**, particularly those genes that differentiate cells related to male sexual function and maturation. One such function is to regulate the growth, development and maintenance of the prostate gland.

A reminder is in order on the importance of gene expression and how it works. The central dogma of biology is that DNA is transcribed to messenger RNA, which is translated to proteins. This schematically is written as:

DNA ➔ mRNA ➔ proteins.
(The Central Dogma of Biology)

DNA is the code, messenger RNA is the vehicle in which the code is transported away from the crowded confines of

DNA, and protein is the output and is the "stuff" of our bodies. Proteins are workhorses of life and include enzymes, chemical transporters/receptors, structural components, and defense components (of the immune system).

All proteins are coded in genes that are just segments of the body's DNA in each cell. The AR is itself a protein; but what it does is to bind with DNA to coax it to activating certain genes to transcribe RNA. This is called expressing the gene. Ultimately the RNA is translated into proteins, a different protein for each gene. Some of these proteins are for the cell to proliferate and grow, which of course for a cancer cell we do not wish to occur.

Findings In a Nutshell

The major scientific findings of the 2004 UCLA work is that the molecular transition of hormone sensitive prostate cancer to hormone insensitive cancer is an increase in mRNA and in the number of androgen receptors expressed. Stated differently, a cancer cell begins to produce more androgen receptors, which then promotes expression of a long list of genes promoting cell growth and replication. The terminology used until then of "hormone refractory" is simply the wrong concept. The problem now is that even a tiny amount of androgen will find a willing androgen receptor to bind with, which produces Trouble. I'll use the term refractory somewhat below in keeping with the terminology and thinking of that time. We now use the term castrate resistant prostate cancer (CRPC).

This is curious and seems paradoxical, in view of the fact that these patients are androgen deprived. More androgen receptors would suggest that there is more androgen around to bind to and activate the AR. But it is likely that with an increase in ARs, there are finally enough to pick up even the smallest amount of androgen still floating around, and thus fueling the cancer. However, is the increased mRNA coding for the AR protein just a symptom of the cancer's refractory behavior or is it the cause?

The major finding of the UCLA group and collaborators are these:

1. First, and most important, it is the androgen receptor that is implicated in the transition from androgen sensitive to androgen independent (refractory or castrate resistant) prostate cancer cells. It is critical to know that the AR is still active when prostate cancer progresses and moves down the progression spiral and becomes refractory. Knowing what the culprit is allows us develop our own tricks to stop it from occurring. That is, if we are smart enough and put resources into it.

2. The cause of progression is an increase in the number of androgen receptors produced in the PCa cells. The ARs are not different when the cancer is refractory compared to when it is androgen dependent. There are just more of them, about three times more. Like mighty armies, large numbers become powerful.

3. The number of androgen receptors must increase for progression to occur. If the number of receptors is decreased, the progression does not move forward.

4. Activation of the androgen receptor occurs by binding to ligands. A ligand is a molecule that binds to another molecule, and in this case the ligands are androgens like DHT and testosterone. Thus ligands are still needed even when the cancer cells become hormone refractory.

5. Androgen receptor meditated cancer progression occurs by the AR traveling to the cell nucleus and binding to DNA. We now know that the AR acts by activating the expression of androgen driven genes. The importance of this finding is that nothing has changed in the action of the AR. It is acting in the same way before and after the cell becomes androgen refractory.

6. The behavior of antiandrogen drugs like Bicalutamide is very different when the cell becomes refractory. Cancer never stops with its deviousness. The increase of AR levels change antagonists to agonists. This means that drugs that were our friends become foe. Anti-androgens like Bicalutamide inhibit the AR and are called antagonists since they inhibit the action of the AR. They fill up the binding spot that androgens use to bind to the AR, which results in

activation of the AR. When the cancer cells change from androgen dependent to refractory, anti-androgens stop inhibiting the AR and become traitors; they start to help the AR do its job. Bicalutamide, which suppress the AR, can become **stimulants** for the prostate cancer cells once they are androgen refractory. The reason this occurs is that antiandrogens begin to help assemble other players (coactivators and corepressors) to the genes that the AR targets for expression. Additionally, there are plenty of ARs around, so blocking them all is no longer effective.

The Bottom Line of This Work

When a prostate cancer cell changes from hormone sensitive to hormone refractory there is an increase in the number of AR receptors in the cells. The increase is substantial, a 3- to 5- fold increase, but the increase is not over the top as might first be expected from a runaway cancer cell.

The reasons for all these events occurring are not crystal clear because high AR levels affect other molecular factors. Excess AR produces an upset in the balance of other molecular factors that control and inhibit gene expression of androgen related genes. Knowing this leads to new opportunities for intervention.

One important discovery is that binding of an androgen to the ligand-binding domain (a specific region of the AR protein) must occur for disease progression. Although we should not mess with Texas, perhaps we can mess with the ligand-binding domain to stop the disease. (Enter Enzalutamide; Chapter 4.)

There are other potential places we can mess with. It is found that it is necessary for the AR to translocate from the cytoplasm to the nucleus. The cytoplasm is the outer region of the cell, and the nucleus is the inner core of the nucleus where DNA resides. This suggests a potential drug therapy that attaches to the AR that stops the translocation.

Disease progression actually occurs by the binding of the AR to form an complex of two ARs in a complex on the

DNA. Is there a drug that targets the AR complex DNA binding region that messes up the ability to bind? (Enter Bromodomain inhibitors; Chapter 17.) Related to this, one can imagine a drug therapy that inhibits the assembly of the pair of ARs. (That is stop formation of the AR transcription complex.)

Some of the new discoveries since 2010 directly or indirectly are related to the androgen receptor. Abiraterone acetate works by reducing the synthesis of androgens, so that androgens never get to the androgen receptor and cannot activate it. Enzalutamide prevents the binding of androgens to the androgen receptor.

What Is This Androgen Receptor Anyway?

A protein is a molecule, which is in the form of a long chain of amino acids. The human body uses twenty different amino acids and a protein consists of a string of them like a string of pearls. But unlike a string of pearls, the amino acids attract or repel each other so that the string folds up into a complex shape; this gives it amazing functional powers. As they say in biology, **form is function**.

The AR is just such a chain of amino acids, which is a protein. AR is a nuclear receptor, of 3 domains (regions).
* An N-terminal variable domain
* A highly conserved DNA binding domain
* A conserved ligand binding domain (LBD).
Conserved means most us (and other species such as chimps) have the same amino acid sequence.

Figure 3-1 shows a cartoon of the ligand-binding domain of the human androgen receptor. The dominant substructures are the helical shapes of the string called alpha helices. There are eleven of them. But the critical region is the ligand-binding pocket where the free-floating androgen eventually settles into. This rendering from an X-ray crystallographic experiment shows a testosterone molecule bound in the pocket. The pocket is very selective. Only very specific molecules like testosterone and DHT will fit and stay there. But that also means if we find another good fitting molecule, we can block out androgens. Once androgen enters the binding pocket, it activates the AR. Minor modifications of ligand structure have a great impact on the strength of interaction.

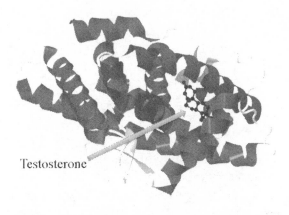

Testosterone

Figure 3-1. Ribbon diagram of the amino acid chain of the ligand-binding domain of the AR. The natural fold produces a pocket where androgens, like testosterone, bind. Structure determined from x-ray crystallography by K. Pereira et al., Protein Science **15**, 987-999 (2006).

The cell has an inner portion called the nucleus where the cell's DNA lays protected, and outside the nucleus is the cytoplasm. The binding of an androgen such as testosterone occurs in the cytoplasm of the cell. The progression is schematically as follows (L=Ligand):

Free L & AR → L,AR (cytoplasm)   [Step 1]
→ translocates   [Step 2]
→ $(L,AR)_2$ → $(L,AR)_2$ + DNA (nucleus). [Step 3]

A schematic of the main steps are shown in **Figure 13-2**. In step 1, the ligand (for example testosterone) and the AR are free floating in the cytoplasm. The ligand binds to the AR in the cytoplasm and form an (L,AR) complex. In step 2, the (L,AR) complex translocates from the cytoplasm to the nucleus. In step 3, two complexes bind together to form a pair (a dimer), and the dimer binds with DNA other factors attached to DNA. It binds to androgen response elements, which are regulator regions of genes that respond to the AR. The final DNA binding provides the signal to recruit machinery in the cell nucleus to express that gene. Expressing the gene means the cell is following the central dogma of biology, DNA => mRNA => protein, with the proteins being formed that were coded by the DNA, and selectively chosen by the AR.

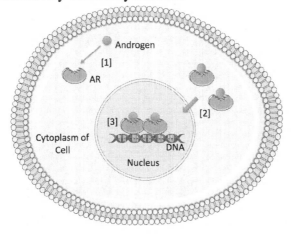

Figure 3-2. A schematic of androgen activation of the androgen receptor (AR) to express androgen responsive genes carried on DNA. The major steps are [1] androgen (ligand) binding to the AR in the outer region of the cell, [2] androgen+AR passing through the membrane of the nucleus where DNA resides, and [3] binding of a pair of androgen+AR complexes to DNA causing genes to be expressed and cell growth and reproduction.

The Experiments

It is very informative to see what experiments were performed, how they were done, and how the pieces of the puzzle came together. Additionally, this experimental bag of tricks is used in most cancer research, so understanding at some level these experiments helps us to understand the larger body of work.

The 2004 experiments were of two main types. 1) Gene profiling and 2) mice models of cancer growth.

Gene profiling. The goal here is to find out what goes on in a prostate cancer cell when it transforms from androgen sensitive to refractory. Cancer is devious, but sometimes we get a break. There could have been many genes that change their expression levels significantly in the transition, but our break is that there is predominantly just one—the gene that expresses the androgen receptor. A hungry detective corners her suspect, and the suspect is the AR.

The tool used is called a DNA microarray. Its name suggests a more complicated device than it really is. In physical shape it is a microscope slide, a 1 inch by 3 inch piece of glass, but on it is a set of grid boxes, and there may be thousands of these grid boxes. Each grid box is an address, a little like a computer memory storage, but chemical instead of electrical. Within each address are thousands of identical fragments of single stranded DNA of known sequence, such as ... ATTAGGCCA.... If we were to place another single strand of DNA in this address that had a complementary sequence to the fragment, it would stick. Recall that "A" only sticks to "T" and vice versa and that "G" only sticks to "C" and vice versa. For instance if we have a DNA fragment of ATTAGGCCA in that address, then any single stranded DNA gene that we wish to uncover that had within it the sequence TAATCCGGT will stick (hybridize) to the address. We know what each address contains because it was constructed commercially with a known sequence. We know the sequence of our genes, for example the gene for the AR. What we want to know is if our target gene (for example the AR gene) is being expressed. When a sample of DNA sticks to an address, we learn what a part of the sequence of that DNA sample is, because we know what is at that address. Colored dyes (described below) will indicate when sticking occurs. The goal is to put all this information together to determine if the AR gene, and other genes, is being expressed. Comparisons can be made between normal prostate cells, hormone sensitive PCa cells, and hormone refractory PCa cells.

The DNA of the cancer cells is not taken directly from the cells. Rather it is taken from the messenger RNA (mRNA). When a gene is expressed in the cell, it creates mRNA. Recall the central dogma of biology: DNA is transcribed to mRNA, and then translated into protein. So by collecting mRNA in the cell, we are being told by the cell what proteins (enzymes, receptors, transporters etc.) it is making. We get a snapshot at that time as to what business the cell is up to. Of particular relevance here, we compare androgen sensitive cells to androgen refractory cells to determine differences. This is the key idea in sorting out what causes the transition from androgen sensitive to castrate resistant prostate cancer.

RNA (or mRNA) does not have the same 4 bases as DNA so it will not stick to a DNA sequence on the microarray. This little setback is overcome by using a reverse transcriptase enzyme, which runs part of the central dogma in reverse — it transcribes mRNA into DNA instead of the other way around. The DNA that is created is then cut into fragments, compatible with the size of the addresses. Enzymes do the cutting.

The next hurdle is to know when something sticks to an address. A colored dye, such as red, is attached to each DNA fragment created by the reverse transcriptase so that it fluoresces (glows) when light is shone upon it. Tersely put, it lights up red. Let's look at the specific address containing ATTAGGCCA. If the target DNA fragment does not have the sequence TAATCCGGT in it, it will not stick and that address does not light up and is black. It if does, then that address lights up red. We get a yes (red) or no (black) answer from the many addresses. Since we know the DNA sequence of the genes such as that of the AR (that's what mapping the human genome is all about), we can determine which genes the cell is expressing.

But there is a wrinkle. Cells express thousands of genes, so this is getting more complex than need be. The question is rephrased to this: "What is the difference in expression levels of genes in a hormone sensitive cancer cell and a hormone refractory cell?" This makes the analysis far easier and more direct.

We make two sets of samples. One set comes from androgen sensitive cells and the other from the refractory cells. But we attach different colored dyes to them; say one green (androgen sensitive) and the other red (androgen refractory). The samples are then pooled together and the mass is applied to the microarray. Instead of two possibilities (black or red as before) each address can yield four possibilities, green, red, yellow or black. They are (i) green (more of or only androgen sensitive), red (more of or only androgen refractory), yellow (both androgen sensitive and refractory attach), or black (neither attach). Since we know what is in each address, we can see what differences there are between the two types of cancer cells.

Mice models. The prostate cancer cells used were from seven different cell lines used in prostate cancer research. The cells were placed in mice. The fact that human cells are placed in mice is called a xenograft, grafting cells from one species into another. Castrated mice led eventually to hormone refractory cancer tumors.

There were 12,559 different genes being tested. To do all this, the thousands of pieces of information require numerical processing algorithms on a computer. The microarray data is scanned using a laser.

The astonishing result is that only one gene was expressed differently between androgen sensitive and refractory prostate cancer cells in all seven cell lines. And that of course was for the androgen receptor. We've found our suspect, and he is holding a smoking gun.

A Closer Look

The androgen receptor is expressed more in castrate resistant PCa. What is cause and what is effect? Perhaps resistance is caused by something else, but produces more AR as a side effect.

We can artificially increase the number of AR within the cell by infecting the cells with a retrovirus. A retrovirus infection causes the DNA of the virus to be inserted into the host. A retrovirus was engineered to insert its DNA into a human cancer cell line that was sensitive to hormones. The engineered DNA contained the gene for the AR. The infected cells produced a 3x amount of AR compared to a control group without the retroviral DNA. The 3x is similar to the microarray results. The cells were then inserted into mice.

The result of these experiments show that only about half the amount of time is needed to develop tumors in mice with AR-over-expressing prostate cancer cells compared to "normal" prostate cancer cells. So just having more AR's produced in the cell is enough to cause a rapid increase in the rate of prostate cancer progression. This approximate 2-fold increase in the tumor formation rate occurred even in castrated mice. As a matter of information, over-expression of the AR need not only come from a single gene being turned on more frequently (that is, being expressed more often), but also by aberrations of the cell's DNA that has changed so that the AR gene is amplified, meaning it has multiple copies of the AR gene.

Cells were also grown in a test tube. Cells that over expressed ARs grew at androgen levels just 20% of needed for androgen sensitive cells. This is not a surprise, as less androgen is needed if there are more receptors to grab whatever there is. But they still needed androgen. Cutting off androgen is still a viable therapy.

We've seen that increasing AR expression leads to disease progression. But is it necessary for disease progression, or is it just accelerating what would happen anyway?

A second retrovirus is used to infect refractory cancer cells. This virus sends out an RNA that causes a reduction in the level of AR expression in the cells, a so-called knockdown process. Mice that were knocked-down implanted with the AR reducing cell grew tumors at a rate that was about one fifth that of the unknocked-down mice. But what is most impressive is that cells that escaped the viral knockdown process produced the tumors that did grow from the knocked-down mice. This is known because the knockdown process was designed to also include a green fluorescent protein that gives color to a knockdown cell. The tumors were not colored.

It takes two to tango. Just the presence of increased AR is not enough for disease progression. There must be a ligand to attach to the AR for the deadly tango to begin. What needs to be shown is that cells expressing increased levels of AR that do not bind ligands do not progress the disease just by themselves. They must have another chemical (an androgen) that binds to them for the disease to progress. It amounts to asking what sounds like a stupid question: Are androgens needed for the disease to progress when the disease is in the "androgen independent" regime?

The answer is yes! When androgen independent, the ARs still needs androgen. It is better to refer to them as androgen-resistant. To progress, the PCa cells must be scavenging the small amounts of androgen around even when androgen levels are very small. Or they are making it themselves.

In order to show that ligand binding is necessary, single point mutations of the androgen receptor were made. This was accomplished by mutating ever so slightly the amino acid sequence in the AR protein. Simply changing one amino acid in the long chain of them can make a difference if it is in the right place. The AR protein folds up in a specific way (**Figure 3-1**), and one region, the ligand-binding domain, is where ligands (androgens) attach. The attachment activates the AR to do its job. A mutation in the binding domain reduces the chance of an androgen binding to the AR.

Two separate single mutations were constricted and both reduced the binding significantly, but not entirely. The two mutants were in cells producing high AR levels (castrate-resistant). The experiments were done in test tubes. The mutant cells were compared to cells with high AR producing cells (also castrate resistant) that were not mutated, and compared to un-mutated cells with low AR numbers (castrate sensitive). The growth of mutated cells occurred far more slowly than the growth of un-mutated cells, and this was true if the un-mutated cells were castrate-resistant or not.

All of this points to the need for androgen to activate the cells—lower the chance of androgen binding by reducing the number of AR receptors or reducing the affinity of an androgen to bind to the AR reduces the progression of the disease. The conclusions so far are that disease progression to hormone resistance is produced by an increase in a cell's ability to express androgen receptors, and that androgen receptors still need androgen, in very low amounts, for the cancer to progress. There is no such animal, at least at this part of our story, as androgen independent progression. Unfortunately, later we will see that mutated ARs (such as AR-V7 splice variants) can truly be androgen independent.

Androgen Receptor Meditated Progression is Genotropic

Genotropic means that cancer progression by the androgen receptor occurs only when the AR makes its way into the cell nucleus, home of the genome carrying DNA. The next set of experiments is designed to determine how the activated AR works.

What is found is that the in order for the cell to grow uncontrollably, the activated AR cannot stay in the cytoplasm. It is conceivable that it could just direct other molecules, proteins or signaling molecules to activate the cell. It is found that the activated AR in the cytoplasm of the cell must leave. It must pass through (translocate) the central core of the cell into the nucleus. This is where the DNA is. It then binds to the nucleus and signals the cell to grow/replicate. Clearly this suggests another target. Stop the translocation — inhibit disease progression.

How do we know all that the AR must translocate? Experiments were performed with cells that were engineered to not have a nuclear localization signal; this prevents translocation of the AR. They were grown in a test tube in low androgen medium. Comparing the growth of these cells, which are castrate resistant, to regular castrate resistant cells, shows a large reduction of cell growth comparable to non-castrate resistant cells, also in low androgen conditions. The cells need to enter the nucleus to activate the cell to progress. In addition a mutant with a single amino acid change that reduces binding to DNA similarly reduced the growth.

The AR must get inside the nucleus to cause harm. But what does it do there? Androgen receptors attach to certain genes within the DNA to do their job. But there is much more involved to gene expression than just attachment. Other molecules, called "factors," must be recruited to the site for the gene to be expressed. The enzyme RNA polymerase must also bind and does the actual transcription. Recall the central dogma of biology. The enzyme (protein) polymerase is the machine to read the DNA and make (transcribe) a new molecule of RNA, which has the same information as the DNA, but it is mobile. It is a messenger to be read later by another enzyme which will translate that code to produce the protein encoded by the original gene within DNA. An example of the process is the kallikrein-3 gene. This gene codes for prostate specific antigen (PSA). When this gene is expressed (DNA => RNA => protein), the PSA protein is created and can be found in blood serum. We monitor the blood serum levels of PSA since it tells us if the

AR is actively expressing genes. Levels of this protein in blood serum are what we think about and worry about often.

So what does high levels of AR do to affect gene expression like PSA? To answer this, experiments were performed that takes apart DNA with its attaching factors while genes are being expressed. The experiment is called chromatin immunoprecipitation, or ChIP for short. Chromatin is a large molecular complex that DNA wraps around in the nucleus; a sort of storage medium. ChIP experiments give a kind of snapshot of which genes on the DNA are attracting attention in that cell. What the ChIP experiments found is that high androgen receptor levels alter the factors that are being bound to DNA. And there are several of these. One example is particularly striking. An androgen, such as DHT, will recruit the AR and RNA polymerase to the DNA. This is just what would be expected. Androgen causes the AR to be activated, which translocates to the DNA then encourages polymerase to come along and start expressing the genes by making RNA.

The action of Bicalutamide is quite surprising. Bicalutamide is a standard antiandrogen given in ADT to patients with hormone sensitive PCa. Bicalutamide is an antagonist (inhibits) by attaching to the AR so androgen cannot bind to the AR. This helps to halt the action of the AR. Some androgen is still able to bind since androgens have a strong affinity for the AR, but much of the trouble is arrested. A comparison of the action of Bicalutamide is made between hormone sensitive and hormone refractory PCa cells. In hormone sensitive cells it is found that without androgen like DHT, bicalutamide acting on the AR produces a recruitment of the AR to DNA, but polymerase is not recruited. The AR is not activated enough to promote the attachment of RNA polymerase. Thus transcription of RNA cannot be made. However, in cells over-expressing AR, (refractory) cells with Bicalutamide alone without androgen can recruit both the AR and RNA polymerase to DNA. There are other factors that are recruited as well when there are high AR levels.

Bicalutamide has other effects in refractory cells. Refractory cells increase the number of androgen receptors that they produce, so it seems logical then to increase the dose of Bicalutamide to counter this. Cells that were infected with the retrovirus that increase AR expression are compared with the same cells but infected with a harmless virus (infecting with the coloring protein GFP). This experiment mimics a comparison between refractory and hormone sensitive PCa cells. The expression of the hormone sensitive cells had the usual response PSA response to Bicalutamide — more Bicalutamide less expression of PSA protein. The refractory cells expressed PSA quite differently. There was little expression at low Bicalutamide levels, but at very high concentration PSA expression increase rapidly. It not unique to Bicalutamide; Flutamide responded similarly. The antagonist (blocker) becomes a weak agonist (enhancer) at high doses — our ally has become our enemy.

The lesson here is that high androgen receptor levels produce a cascade of other events which are not fully understood, but lead to chemical changes that alter the supply of factors that influence gene expression. This altered cocktail produces different behavior with Bicalutamide. Second generation antiandrogens (blockers) are needed.

Some Remarks

The discovery that the androgen receptor is still an important player even in castrate resistant prostate cancer is truly amazing. It changes our thinking on how prostate cancer progresses, and it produces hope that similar advances (soon) will do the same. One can't also help but feel that the answer lies in research and major developments are just around the corner — that we are at a cusp in our understanding of how to remedy this disease. But the research has to be inspired, producing revolution and not evolution, and removing misconceptions like PCa being androgen independent when advanced to CRPC. We need the right research; maybe I should call it "better" research. Better does not necessarily mean more.

References

(UCLA) Molecular determinants of resistance to antiandrogen therapy, CD Chen, DS Welsbie, C Tran, SH Baek, R Chen, R Vessella, MG Rosenfeld and CL Sawyers, Nature Medicine 10(1), 33-39 (2004).

Comparison of crystal structures of human androgen receptor ligand-binding domain completed with various agonists reveals molecular determinants responsible for binding affinity, K. Pereira, D. Jesus-Tran, P-L Cote, L. Cantin, J. Blanch et, F. Labrie, and R. Brenton, Protein Science **15**, 987-999 (2006). The relevant PDB file of the structure is 2AM9 of testosterone in the binding pocket of the AR.

Chapter 4

Quit Grabbing Trouble:
Enzalutamide

Quam continuis et quantis longa senectus/Plena malis!
How incessant and great are the ills with which a prolonged
old age is replete!
Juvenal, Roman poet of the 1ˢᵗ Century.

Enzalutamide is one of the latest weapons to be
added to the arsenal to combat castrate resistant prostate
cancer. The FDA approval occurred on August 31, 2012.
The mechanism of action Enzalutamide (also known as
MDV3100 or XTANDI) is by its interaction with the
androgen receptor (AR). Enzalutamide binds to the AR
filling the space of the binding pocket so that the androgens
testosterone or DHT cannot get in. It competes against
androgens for the binding pocket, and when it fills, it does
not activate the androgen receptor in the same way that
androgens do.
Enzalutamide is a second-generation antiandrogen
that is for patients who have become castration resistant. It is
a small molecule, and not a steroid. This second-generation
anti-androgen follows the first-generation non-steroid
antiandrogens Flutamide, Nilutamide and the very widely
used Bicalutamide. The second-generation Enzalutamide
does not produce agonist activity as the disease wears on to
castrate resistance, as do the first-generation drugs.

Discovery
The discovery of Enzalutamide is a direct
consequence of the discoveries concerning the importance
and behavior of the androgen receptor discussed in Chapter

3. We will go through some of this process, as it is an example of how drug discovery works in prostate cancer research.

The goal is to develop a second-generation antiandrogen, to replace first-generation drugs like Bicalutamide. The work starts with a chemical RU59063 that has a high affinity for the AR (1/3 the affinity of

Figure 4-1. Chemical structure of Enzalutamide (Also known as MDV3100 or Xtandi.) The original work is reported in: C. Tran et al., Science 324 787-790 (2009).

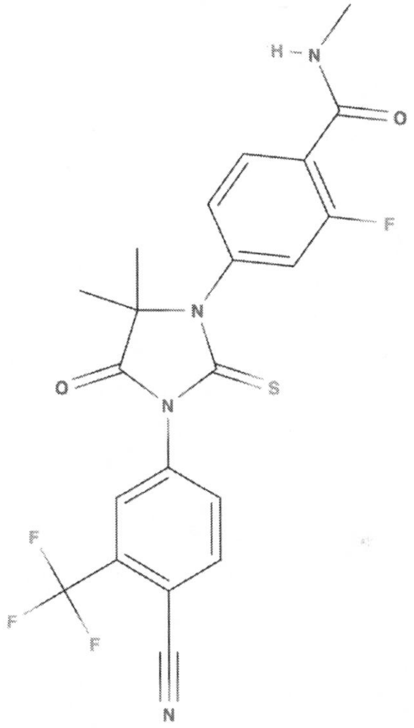

testosterone) and is not selective of other receptors. Then begins a process to screen similar compounds in an iterative process of 200 derivatives. The search is performed in human prostate cells with varying amounts of AR. The procedure led to a US 20070004753 patent.

In the end, two candidates were selected for biological studies — RD162 and MDV3100. MDV31000 was ultimately chosen for human trials based on results from studies in mice and because its drug characteristics where more favorable. MDV3100 (later called Enzalutamide) has a

6 ring, and a 5 ring with nitrogen, another 6 ring, and a tail with N and O. MDV3100 was found to bind to the AR much better than Bicalutamide but less than DHT.

The key to activation is the conformational change of the AR that occurs when a molecule enters the binding pocket. Androgens like DHT and testosterone induce a change of shape of the AR that allows other molecules to bind to the AR and DNA and cause expression of AR targeted genes. The change in conformation with MDV3100 is different, and binding of these co-activator molecules is thwarted.

MDV3100 (Enzalutamide) was found to suppress growth of cells and induces apoptosis (programmed cell death). However, if there is plenty of androgen around (higher than castration levels), androgen will bind more effectively to the AR and will defeat the action of MDV3100.

One of the problems with first generation antiandrogens like Bicalutamide is that they can change from friend to foe. When PCa cells begin to over-express AR as it ramps up aggressiveness, Bicalutamide changes from an antagonist to an agonist. This means instead of inactivating cells it activates them to stimulate genes such as PSA and transmembrane serine protease 2 (TMPRSS2). MDV3100 did not do this.

Does It Work? The Evidence.

The first clinical trial for Enzalutamide was for patients that had already underwent chemotherapy with taxanes (Docetaxel). The trial was successful, which again shows that the androgen receptor is still active and that prostate cancer cells are not resistant to hormones — they still need them to be active. It is more like they become hormone hypersensitive prostate cancer cells. A second recent trial is underway for earlier stage prostate cancer patients, specifically for those that have not yet undergone chemotherapy. This led to FDA approval in 2014 for mCRPC before taxanes.

The discovery of Enzalutamide is a remarkable advance. There is more to Enzalutamide than one would expect at first glance. It acts in multiple ways, and the three main modes of action are that Enzalutamide (i) prevents binding of androgens to the AR, (ii) it prevents the AR from translocating to the nucleus, and (iii) it inhibits binding of the AR with DNA and the recruitment of other activator agents (co-activator) that enable expression of genes. Recall that the androgen receptor is activated by androgens, passes (translocates) from the cytoplasm to the nucleus where the DNA is stored, and binds to the DNA at androgen-controlled genes to grow or produce new cells. Overall, Enzalutamide is an androgen receptor signaling inhibitor.

The other androgen pathway drug is Abiraterone Acetate, which works in a different way. Abiraterone acts by inhibiting the synthesis of testosterone and DHT. Enzalutamide prevents androgens from activating the AR, while Abiraterone prevents the production of "fuel" for the AR. Thus the two drugs, Enzalutamide and Abiraterone Acetate, work in complementary and hopefully not cross-reacting ways to shut down the action of the AR. However, there is some cross-resistance between these two drugs.

Unfortunately most good things come to an end. The big disappointment of Enzalutamide is that most patients eventually become resistant to it. The AR is over-expressed within prostate cancer cells allowing extremely low levels of androgen to activate the cell. Activation leads to cell growth of the aggressive cancer cells. Prostate cancer cells also mutate so that weaker androgens can cause the cell to be activated. And finally, PCa cells can produce their own androgens (autocrine production) so that they need no external stimulus — they active themselves.

Enzalutamide works on the androgen receptor pathway that activates cells to grow. For this therapy to work, the AR must still control the disease. Thus Enzalutamide will not be effective for everyone, and it is difficult to determine who will or will not respond. Enzalutamide can potentially be used with Abiraterone,

Docetaxel, Cabazitaxel, Ra223, or immunotherapy. Which combinations to use and in which order is a matter of serious debate.

The first clinical trial of Enzalutamide that was started in 2009 was the AFFIRM trial. This trial of Enzalutamide had about 1200 men enrolled and led to increased survival, the gold standard of positive results. This led to FDA approval in 2012 for metastatic CRPC who had already been administered Docetaxel. When the trial started Docetaxel (chemo) was effectively the end of the line for treatments. But during the trial, Cabazitaxel (a chemo drug now usually given after Docetaxel) and Abiraterone Acetate with Prednisone were approved.

Recall that castration resistance is caused primarily by an increase in the number of androgen receptors in the prostate cancer cell. This allows very low levels of androgens to fuel the development of prostate cancer cells. This study then was to inhibit the action of these AR overproducing cells.

The study was a double blind where neither the researchers nor the patients knew which group they were in — the Enzalutamide group or the placebo group. Two thirds were in the Enzalutamide group and one third in the placebo group.

The results are encouraging as determined by the median time of survival. The median time of survival is the amounts of time after taking the drug that one-half of the patients survive. Unfortunately, this also means that one-half of the patients have died. Those on the Enzalutamide group had a median time of survival of 18.4 months, while those on the placebo had a median time of survival of 13.6 months, thus it increased survival by 4.8 months. Of course PCa sufferers are looking for years or decades of increased survival, not months. But it's a start; a slow one.

Prostate cancer patients carefully monitor their serum PSA levels. PSA levels were cut more than in half in 54% of men, while only 2% of the placebo group achieved this. It's a pity that such drastically reductions of PSA did not lead to drastic survival times. PSA levels are not perfect indicators.

There were some modest increases in relatively minor adverse effects with the Enzalutamide group compared to the placebo group. These include fatigue 34% vs. 29%, diarrhea 21% vs. 18%, musculoskeletal pain 14% vs. 10%, and headache 12% vs. 6%. The most significant and serious adverse effect was seizures. No patients had seizures in the placebo group of 399 patients, while 5 had seizures in the Enzalutamide group of 800. The brain has a protective coating called the blood brain barrier that keeps potentially harmful chemicals out. Enzalutamide crosses the blood-brain barrier.

It is hypothesized that many of the side effects were a result of the reduced hormone levels that resulted in the Enzalutamide group, which affects negatively other healthy tissue that uses some level of androgen. More serious adverse effects were lower in the Enzalutamide group than in the placebo group. A likely explanation of this is that the disease progressed more in the placebo group.

The second trial was the Phase III PREVAIL trial (NCT01212991), which was given to men with metastatic prostate cancer before they received Docetaxel. Docetaxel is a first-line chemotherapy, and often is given late in the treatment, as chemotherapy can be tough. The trial period was 2010-2012, and was for mCRPC patients all of which continued androgen deprivation therapy. The patients had not take Abiraterone Acetate. The trial was double blind with 50% receiving Enzalutamide, and 50% a placebo. The study was large with 1,717 men, and key outcomes were radiographic progression free survival (RPFS) and overall survival.

The 12-month outcome was particularly significant. The RPFS results were 65% vs. 14% for the Enzalutamide group and the placebo group respectively. The hazard ratio (HR) of the two groups was 0.19, or about a 5-fold increase in RPFS time in the Enzalutamide group. The overall survival results were 72% vs. 63% for the two groups

64

(Enzalutamide vs. placebo). For those with soft-tissue metastases, there was a complete partial response of 59% for the Enzalutamide group, but only 5% in the placebo group.

The median duration of patients within the trial was only 22 months and the overall survival time was longer than this. This means that only estimates of median overall survival time can be made. The results for median overall survival times are 32.4 months vs. 30.2 months for the Enzalutamide and placebo groups respectively. This is disappointing in that there is only a 2.2-month median increase in survival time. Enzalutamide appears to delay progression at first, which is worth much, but eventually it catches up with not a large increase in overall survival time. These are estimates. Let's hope that the true increase is longer.

References

Enzalutamide: Looking back at its preclinical discovery, YS Ha and K IY, Expert Opinion Drug Discovery, 12, 1-9 (2014).

Increased Survival with Enzalutamide in Prostate Cancer after Chemotherapy, HI Scher, K Fizazi, F Saad, M-E Taplin, CN Sternberg, K Miller, R de Wit, P Mulders, KN Chi, Neal D. Shore, AJ Armstrong, TW Flaig, A Fléchon, P Mainwaring, M Fleming, JD Hainsworth, M Hirmand, B Selby, L Seely, and JS de Bono, for the AFFIRM Investigators, New England Journal of Medicine 367, 1187-1197 (2012).

Enzalutamide in Metastatic Prostate Cancer before Chemotherapy, TM Beer, AJ Armstrong, DE Rathkopf, Y Loriot, CN Sternberg, CS Higano, P Iversen, S Bhattacharya, J Carles, S Chowdhury, ID Davis, JS de Bono, CP Evans, K Fizazi, AM Joshua, C-S Kim, G Kimura, P Mainwaring, H Mansbach, K Miller, SB Noonberg, F Perabo, D Phung, F Saad, HI Scher, M-E Taplin, PM Venner, and B Tombal, for the PREVAIL Investigators, The New England Journal of Medicine, 371(5), 424-33 (2014).

Development of a Second-Generation Antiandrogen for Treatment of Advanced Prostate Cancer, C Tran, S Ouk, NJ Clegg, Y Chen, PA Watson, V Arora, J Wongvipat, PM Smith-Jones, D Yoo, A Kwon, T Wasielewska, D Welsbie, C Degui Chen, CS Higano, TM Beer, David T. Hung, Howard I. Scher, ME Jung, CL Sawyers, Science **324**, 787 (2009).

Chapter 5

Stop Making Trouble: Abiraterone Acetate

[I]gnorance more frequently begets confidence than does knowledge. Charles Darwin

The androgen receptor numbers can explode in castrate resistant prostate cancer. These large numbers of receptors seek out and bind to scarce quantities of androgens in patients on androgen deprivation therapy. Abiraterone acetate is a drug that is capable of further reducing the concentration of androgens in prostate cancer cells. It does this by interfering with the pathway that synthesizes the androgens testosterone and DHT from other steroids. Abiraterone acetate is the drug taken, but it is not the functional drug. Abiraterone acetate (trade name Zytiga) is a "prodrug" which is converted to abiraterone in the body.

What Does Abiraterone Do?

Abiraterone inhibits a certain enzyme, CYP17A1, that acts on precursor steroids before they become androgens. This enzyme performs two important functions in the pathway to produce testosterone and DHT from other steroids. These two enzymatic functions are hydroxylase and lyase activity. That is an obtuse answer, but as we will see, it is quite understandable and lets us think about other ways we can inhibit these pesky androgens that feed the androgen receptor that promote the growth and division of prostate cancer cells.

In this chapter we will explore some of the chemistry of androgen formation from steroids, and discover how the androgen synthesis can be blocked.

Castration levels of testosterone do not mean there is no testosterone in blood serum, but only that it is very low, less than say 10-20ng/dL. The testes are the primary producer of testosterone, and LHRH agonists (antagonists) largely turned off their production. But there are sources outside the testes (extragonadel). A lesser, but important, source of androgen is the adrenal gland. Even more sinister is the production of androgens within the tumor itself. When cells make hormones for themselves this is referred to as intracrine production. As we will discuss below, steroids such as cholesterol or progesterone or pregnenolone are the raw materials that can be converted by a circuitous pathway into testosterone or DHT final products. The net result is that in the microenvironment of the cancer lesion, there is enough testosterone to activate the androgen receptors. Of course, activating the AR means that the AR will bind to the DNA in the nucleus and cause specific genes to be expressed. These specific genes result in the growth and proliferation of the cancer tumor.

Chemistry And Steroids For Making Testosterone and DHT

Steroids are a class of chemical compounds with a core and attachments. The core consists of four carbon rings fused together. Three of the rings are 6-rings and the fourth ring is a five-member ring. There are 19 carbon atoms in the rings or attached to them, and much of the action occurs in carbon atom number 17. Carbon number 17 is a pivotal atom and can have a variety of attachments that change the name, function, and properties of the steroid. **Figure 5-1** shows the pathway of steroid synthesis from cholesterol (top, left) -and the cholesterol molecule has the carbon atoms numbered. As examples, testosterone has an OH (oxygen, hydrogen) group attached to carbon 17, progesterone has a hydrogen and an O=C-CH3 group attached to it.

We will need to understand chemical figures to fully appreciate the pathway figure. Reading chemical figures is actually very easy. The most important organic chemistry elements are CHON (carbon, hydrogen, oxygen

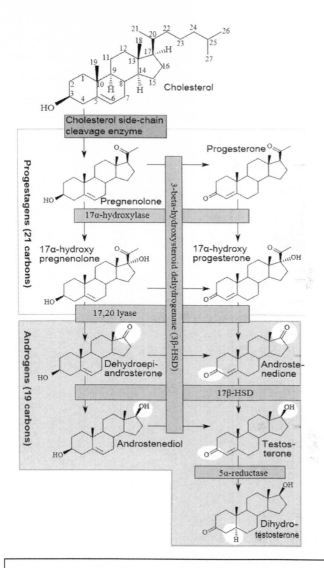

Figure 5-1. Pathways showing the action of various enzymes to produce steroids, including androgens testosterone and dihydrotestosterone from cholesterol (top-left of figure). Note in particular the action of the enzyme activity 17α-hydroxylase and 17,20 lyase, and that of 5alpha-reductase. (Adapted from M Häggström M and D Richfield, Diagram of the pathways of human steroidogenesis, Wikiversity Journal of Medicine 1 (1) (2014).)

and nitrogen). The premier element is carbon, and in chemical figures carbon atoms are not labeled (usually). Nitrogen and Oxygen are always labeled. Carbon is always assumed to have four bonds that connect it to other atoms. A line indicates a bond, so each carbon has four lines connected to it. Some bonds are double bonds and are indicated by two lines, like $O=C=O$ (CO_2, carbon dioxide). If carbon is seen with three bonds or less, then it is assumed that the unseen bonds are single hydrogen atoms. Hydrogen atoms can only form one bond and decorate carbon atoms. Hydrogen so often decorate the structure that we often just do not show them, but the unseen ones are easy to recognize by mentally adding the missing bonds to make the required four for carbon.

Figure 5-1 shows the pathways of the synthesis of various steroids from cholesterol. Steroids often have the suffix -one, like testosterone, and progesterone, or -ide. We will be concentrating on the left vertical pathways of the figure, which ultimately lead to testosterone and dihydrotestoterone (DHT). An enzyme is the molecular machine that accomplishes the changes from one chemical in the pathway to the next. Enzymes are special proteins that are molecular scissors, molecular staplers, or a variety of molecular machines. Often in the chemical literature they are symbolized as a molecular "pac-man" that chomp at bonds cutting them (scissors). But they can add atoms or molecular fragments as well (staplers). Enzymes are proteins, and they are encoded in the cell's DNA and are expressed as needed.

If we look at the last step of the pathway, we see that testosterone is converted to DHT by the enzyme 5-alpha reductase. Note that the suffix –ase is often used to indicate an enzyme. DHT has a far higher affinity for the androgen receptor-binding pocket, thus it is five times more effective in activating the AR than testosterone is. That is why we wish to have DHT levels reduced to as low levels as we can. That is the purpose of 5-alpha reductase inhibitors (5AR inhibitors), like Proscar and Avodart (Finasteride and Dutasteride).

The most important steps for our purposes here are the 17α-hydroxylase and the 17,20 lyase activities.

As an example of the action of 17α-hydroxylase, note that progesterone is converted to 17α-hydroxyprogesterone. The enzyme works on the pivotal carbon atom number 17. It removes a hydrogen atom –H (not shown, but implied in the figure because we see only 3 bonds on C 17) and replacing it with an –O-H. The OH combination is called a hydroxyl group. A key point here is that one cannot proceed down the pathway from cholesterol, pregnenolone or progesterone to testosterone or DHT without the enzyme acting on it. Thus we have a therapeutic target. Stop the progression down the pathway and we arrest the production of testosterone and DHT. This is one of the targets Abiraterone uses to inhibit the synthesis of androgens.

As another example, the enzymatic activity 17,20 lyase cuts the bond between the pivotal carbon atom 17 and carbon 20 on the side chain of intermediate steroids 17α-hydroxypregnenolone or 17α-hydroxyprogesterone. It converts molecules with 21 carbon atoms to those with 19 carbon atoms, which is the number that testosterone and DHT have. The enzyme's action produces dehydropiandrosterone (DHEA) or androstenedione (AED). The enzyme removes the side chain and the –H attached to it and replaces it with a double bonded oxygen, =O. The 17α-hydroxyprogesterone is so very close to testosterone, only differing in that testosterone has the –H replaced and the =O replaced with –OH. But again, we cannot go further down the pathway to testosterone or DHT without 17,20 lyase acting on steroids. Ahha! Another target that Abiraterone uses to inhibit the formation of testosterone and DHT.

The enzyme that produces the enzymatic action of 17α-hydroxylase and 17,20 lyase activity is an enzyme called Cytochrome P 450 17-Alpha hydroxylase, or CYP17A1 for short. It is predominantly in the adrenal gland. Enzymes catalyze (that is accelerate or enable) many reactions involving steroids and fats. For us here, we are

most concerned with its action in the production of
androgens.

The action of Abiraterone is to inhibit the 17α-
hydroxylase and 17,20 lyase enzyme activity. There are two
places that its inhibiting action is needed — in the adrenal
gland for sure, but surprisingly in the source of our Trouble,
the tumor cells. This intracrine production occurs when cells
(here cancer tumor cells) can produce their own hormones.
The adrenal gland although producing only small amounts of
androgens produces enough to fuel the hypersensitive
castrate resistant cells when they are producing excess AR.

The FDA first approved Abiraterone Acetate (AA)
for late stage prostate cancer in April 2011. The origins of
Abiraterone Acetate as a potential prostate cancer androgen
biosynthesis inhibitor for prostate cancer goes back 16 years
in a study published in 1995 in the Journal of Medicinal
Chemistry. The article was right on target with its title,
"Novel steroid inhibitors of human cytochrome P450$_{17\alpha}$
(17α-hydroxylase-C$_{17,20}$-lyase): Potential agents for the
treatment of prostatic cancer." Chemists searched through
many different molecules and found several candidates, but
identified Abiraterone as being potentially beneficial. The
sad fact is that the drug development process is not fast. The
initial results of the search were reported in 1995 (20 years
ago) and suggested Abiraterone as a potential drug for
prostate cancer.

The molecular structure of Abiraterone Acetate is
shown in the molecular diagram, **Figure 5.2**. There are the 4-
fused rings of a steroid, like testosterone, but it also has an
additional ring attached to C 17. This ring is called pyridyl
and it is all carbon and hydrogen except for an important
single nitrogen atom.

How was it determined that this drug would serve as
a good inhibitor? The first feature is that AA is a steroid with
a core similar to other steroids that the CYP17 enzyme acts
on. Modified steroids are good candidates to be assimilated
into the CYP17 binding-pocket and if we are lucky, they
gum-up the works.

A score is given to each potential inhibitor called IC50. IC stands for "inhibitor concentration" which means the amount of drug needed to have a desired effect. The 50 stands for

Figure 5-2. Molecular structure of Abiraterone Acetate. Abiraterone Acetate, changes to Abiraterone in our body where the O-(C=O)-CH$_3$ tail (left) is replaced by an OH group.

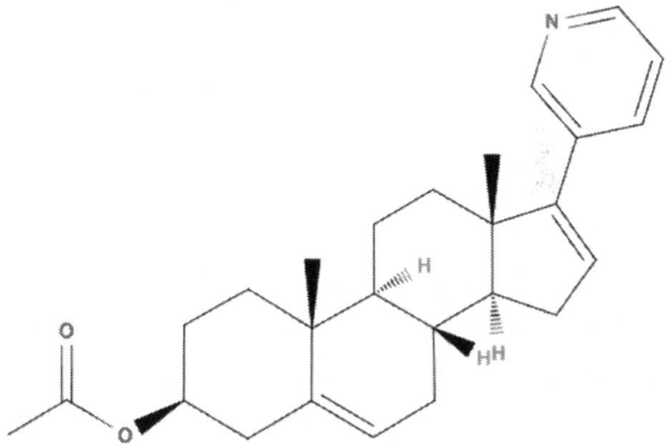

50% inhibition — 50% of the enzymes are inactivated and 50% are not. We want IC50 values that are very small, meaning only a little of the drug is needed. IC50 is what one is referring to when statements are made that one inhibitor is more potent than another. IC50 values of Abiraterone are 2.9nM and 4.0nM for 17,20 lyase and 17α-hydroxylase inhibition respectively. Other drugs tested had IC50 values widely varying with some over 10,000 nM. (nM is nanomolar). The inhibition occurs when abiraterone fits into a pocket of the CYP171A enzyme (**Figure 5-3**), inhibiting its activity.

The key features of Abiraterone that make it work are the nitrogen containing pyridl ring and the conversion of a single bond of carbon 17 in the 5-ring to a double bond. These factors transpire to allow the inhibitor to become engaged within the binding-pocket of the CYP17A1 structure but to keep the molecule from acting on other steroids within the pathway. These scientists were using their intuition. The nitrogen containing pyridl ring was chosen because it is expected to coordinate with a iron atom in an accompanying molecule (cofactor) at an active site of the enzyme. Chemists are often amazing in their ability to "guess" what the right kind of atom or molecule is needed to accomplish a task.

Figure 5-3. Cartoon of the CYP17A1 enzyme with abiraterone (center) bound to it halting CYP17A1's enzymatic activity. Structure from Devore et al., Nature 482, 116 (2012).

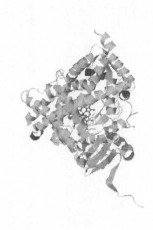

Abiraterone is given with Prednisone. The purpose of Abiraterone is to affect the steroid synthesis pathway, and this can result in the overproduction of mineralolcorticoids (not shown **Figure 5-1**). They are called mineralocorticoids because they affect salt balance (the mineral sodium) and they retain water in the body. Prednisone tempers the development of these mineralolcorticoids. This excess occurred in more than half of the patients. Side effects of this are reduced by Prednisone and include retention of fluid, hypokalemia and a very slight increase in incidence of hypertension.

Clinical Trials

The first phase III clinical trial was the Cougar trial, COU-AA-301, NCT00638690. The trial was sponsored by

Cougar Biotechnology, hence the name. The results appeared in May 2011 in the New England Journal of Medicine in a paper entitled "Abiraterone and Increased Survival in Metastatic Prostate Cancer." There were 1,195 participants in this double blind trial, in a ratio of 2:1 with participants receiving Abiraterone and Prednisone or a placebo and Prednisone. The trial was started in May 2008, with the median time in the trial of about 13 months. These were men who had very advanced castration resistant metastatic prostate cancer and had already gone through chemotherapy with Docetaxel. The goals were to increase overall survival, time to PSA progression, and time of progression-free survival.

All the goals were met favorably. The mean overall survival (mOS) time for the placebo group was 10.9 months, while the Abiraterone group's mOS time was 14.8 months. Median overall survival time increased 3.9 months or 36%. We would like to see a many year increase in OS, but it's a small step in the right direction. Time to PSA progression was also increased in the Abiraterone group (from 6.6 mo to 10.2 mo) as well as progression-free survival (from 3.6 mo to 5.6 mo). All of these outcomes were moderately improved, and it is hoped that these lead to more significant improvements in less progressed patients or when used in combination with other therapies.

The second clinical trial started in April 2009 was for patients with metastatic castrate resistant prostate cancer but earlier on in their treatment and had not yet gone through chemotherapy. The results were published in the New England Journal of Medicine in January 2013, titled "Abiraterone in Metastatic Prostate Cancer without Previous Chemotherapy." The trial, NCT00887198, was funded by Janssen Research and Development, which morphed from Cougar Biotechnology. The trial was a double blind of 1:1 of Abiraterone plus Prednisone vs. a placebo plus Prednisone. The goals were to increase OS and radiographic progression-free survival. The median follow-up time was 22 months. The median overall survival time for the placebo group was

27.2 months, while the median OS for the Abiraterone group was not reached due to the short follow-up time. A rough estimate can be made however from the statistically derived hazard ratio of 0.75. This approximately translates to a 33% increase in overall survival time (9 month increase, from 27.2 mo to 36.2 mo) for those taking Abiraterone. The time of radiographic progression-free survival was 8.3 months for the placebo group and 16.5 months for the Abiraterone group. Thus patients on Abiraterone did not decline as rapidly as those on a placebo, and were able to stay off chemotherapy longer.

Whack a Mole — Trouble Pops Up Somewhere Else

The question naturally arises as to why this is not some sort of permanent cure. First off not all patients respond to Abiraterone, and those that do, most eventually lose the benefits of Abiraterone. It appears that even with the androgen synthesis pathway disrupted, the androgen receptor again begins to signal. Similar to what happens with the failure of ADT where the cells begin producing extreme amounts of androgen receptors, Abiraterone can fail because of an over expression of the CYP17A1 enzyme. Increasing the dosage of Abiraterone is a dicey proposition because other factors also cause Abiraterone to fail. A sinister failure is the appearances of splice variants of the AR. Splice variants are aberrated proteins in which part of their amino-acid sequence is deleted. The AR splice variants will be covered in Chapter 6. Splice variants of the AR can act without the need of any androgen. In this case the blockage of the androgen pathway is no longer relevant. These AR splice variants begin performing the same job previously reserved for androgen activated ARs. Enzalutamide, which works by inactivating the AR by blocking the androgen-binding pocket with the AR, will also not be effective. Splice variants change the entire game.

References

Practical guide to the use of abiraterone in CRPC, EA Mostaghel and DW Lin, Canadian Journal of Urology 21, 57-63 (2014).

Human Cytochrome P450 CYP17A1 in complex with Abiraterone and TOK-001 (Protein data band file 3RUK), NM Devore and EE Scott, Nature 482, 116 (2012).

Abiraterone and Increased Survival in Metastatic Prostate Cancer, JS de Bono et al.,
New England Journal of Medicine 364, 1995-2005 (2011).

Abiraterone in Metastatic Prostate Cancer without Previous Chemotherapy, CJ Ryan et al. (COU-AA-302 investigators), New England Journal of Medicine 368, 138-148 (2013).

Novel steroid inhibitors of human cytochrome P450$_{17\alpha}$ (17α-hydroxylase-C$_{17,20}$-lyase): Potential agents for the treatment of prostatic cancer, GA Potter, SE Barrie, M Jarman and MG Rowlands, Journal of Medicinal Chemistry 38, 2463-2471 (1995).

Chapter 6

Troubling Genes – Mutations, Gene-Fusions, Excess/Reduced Genes, And Other Tricks That Bring On Trouble.

Twenty–first century businesses will rely on American science, technology, research and development. I want the country that eliminated polio and mapped the human genome to lead a new era of medicine—one that delivers the right treatment at the right time. President Barack Obama, Jan. 2015

Basics—From Genes To Proteins

Mutations in DNA are the fundamental cause of cancer. Our DNA is carried in 23 chromosomes, and within these chromosomes lay the genes. Genes are nothing but a particular sequence of the four bases along a strand making the DNA double helix. But the sequence of the four bases carries the code for a protein, like letters carry the code for words or a sentence. Proteins are the active and passive elements within the cell that make it alive. They give the cell its form, its enzymatic activity, its receptors for signaling, its means to transport molecules about, and its defense mechanisms. Proteins with the wrong string of amino acids produced by mutant DNA can produce a diseased or cancerous cell.

DNA contains just four bases, **A, T, G, and C** (adenine, thymine, guanine, and cytosine). The code is similar to Morse Code. In Morse Code the goal is to produce all 26 letters of the alphabet with a series of dots and dashes in different sequences and patterns for each of the 26 letters of the alphabet. From that comes words, then sentences, and with patience an encyclopedia. The DNA code is converted to an RNA code that is read by a nanomachine that makes proteins by sewing together amino acids along a string. The amino-acid string is the protein.

The structure of DNA has been known since the work of Watson and Crick in 1953, as they determined the double helix structure. Pairing a base on one string with a different base on the other connects two strings. The only allowed pairing is A with T and G with C. These are called complementary bases. This lead to an understanding of how genetic material can be copied. As Watson and Crick mention in their one page 1953 paper, "It has not escaped our notice that the specific pairing we have postulated immediately suggests a possible copying of genetic material." When the two strands of the double helix are separated, one can add the complementary bases one at a time to create the other side. Doing this to each original separated strand, produces two complete double helices starting from one.

Watson and Crick did not yet know the actual code from DNA to produce protein. We now know it is a three-letter code, called a codon. Thus a sequence of DNA like AATGCTGAACCTGAA is really AAT GCT GAA CCT GAA. It is like letters forming words. But now what do the words mean? Here is an example of nature's beauty. Nature has figured out that it needs to spell only twenty words. These words are for the twenty amino acids that make a protein. Do not miss the fact that the 4 letters (A, T, G C), when combined into triplets can make 4x4x4=64 different words. Some of the words also say stop and go, to start or stop the amino acid chain. But most of the redundancy is that many different spellings are for the same protein. An example is AGA and CCG both are code for the amino acid Arginine. The DNA string is very long but has start and stop sections for each of the genes that code a protein. It's sort of like a long play list of songs (the DNA), which contains individual songs (the genes to make proteins). An example of the androgen receptor will be given below.

Recall the Central Dogma of biology (Chapter 3); DNA → RNA → Protein. Before DNA is translated into protein, it must first be transcribed into RNA (RiboNucleic Acid). The RNA code is very similar to the DNA code and it has four bases **A, U, G, C** instead of **A, T G, C** in DNA. (Here U is Uracil and replaces T, Thymine, in DNA.) So why bother with creating RNA? DNA is the song-list containing many songs. The RNA sequence is just one song—one specific protein. RNA is small and can be transported around and read easily by protein making enzymes that read the RNA and gather and assemble the amino acids in the correct order to form the protein.

Table 6-1 Amino Acid Name	3 letter abbreviation	Alphabet
Alanine	ALA	A
Arginine	ARG	R
Asparagine	ASN	N
Aspartic acid	ASP	D
Cysteine	CYS	C
Glutamine	GLN	Q
Glutamic acid	GLU	E
Glycine	GLY	G
Histidine	HIS	H
Isoleucine	ILE	I
Leucine	LEU	L
Lysine	LYS	K
Methionine	MET	M
Phenylalanine	PHE	F
Proline	PRO	P
Serine	SER	S
Threonine	THR	T
Tryptophan	TRP	W
Tyrosine	TYR	Y
Valine	VAL	V

There are 20 different amino acids, which can be strung together to make a specific protein. The twenty amino acids are listed **Table 6-1**. Either three letter names or a single letter is used to abbreviate each amino acid. For example TRP or W stands for tryptophan. [As a caution, note that the four DNA bases, A, T, G and C, are NOT at all related to the Alanine (A), Threonine (T), Glycine (G) and Cysteine (C) amino acids.] These twenty building blocks are like the letters for a very long word, the protein. It is not important to know their names. What is important is that drugs and natural processes can seek out specific proteins or seek out certain amino acids, e.g. tyrosine Y, and cause something important to happen. This might be cutting the protein or misfolding it.

Proteins must have the correct sequence of amino acids for them to function properly. But the sequence will be corrupt if the coding DNA is mutated or aberrant. Mutations or aberrations of DNA can be innocuous or all hell can break loose.

Amino acids are strung together in a certain order to make a very long "word" of usually 100-1000 elements long. This ordered long word is a molecule called a protein.

The androgen receptor is just one example of a protein that plays a critical role in our story. The ligand-binding domain of the human androgen receptor protein has 266 amino acids in a string. This is the domain of the androgen receptor that binds androgen (e.g. testosterone) and causes development and growth of PCa cells. The string contains the following amino acid sequence:

```
1                                        40
ETTQKLTVSHIEGYECQPIFLNVLEAIEPGVVCAGHDNNQ
PDSFAALLSSLNELGERQLVHVVKWAKALPGFRNLHVDDQ
MAVIQYSWMGLMVFAMGWRSFTNVNSRMLYFAPDLVFNEY
RMHKSRMYSQCVRMRHLSQEFGWLQITPQEFLCMKALLLF
SIIPVDGLKNQKFFDELRMNYIKELDRIIACKRKNPTSCS
RRFYQLTKLLDSVQPIARELHQFTFDLLIKSHMVSVDFPE
MMAEIISVQVPKILSGKVKPIYFHTQ.
```

You can appreciate the use of a one-letter code to convey information on amino acid content. The sequence of amino acids is Glutamic Acid, Threonine, Threonine, Glutamine, and so on. The DNA sequence that codes for it is three times as long, since each of the 20 amino acids needs a three base codon. For the androgen receptor, the DNA code starts out GAA-ACC-ACC-CAG-... to code for the amino acid sequence ETTQ....

Enough proteins functioning properly constitute the inner working of a cell, and about 30 trillion cells produce one of us.

Finally we are ready to fully appreciate mutations in the DNA sequence. It should now be clear that if the DNA sequence is modified, the proteins they code for might become modified. If they become modified, they may not function properly. Again using the androgen receptor as an example, a mutation could allow the androgen receptor to become activated without the need for androgen.

The simplest mutation is a point mutation, also called single-nucleotide polymorphisms (or SNP). Instead of GAA-ACC-ACC-CAG-... the DNA is mutated to GAA-ACC-ACC-CAC-... This will code for ETTH... instead of ETTQ..., which means instead of a Glutamine in the 4th amino-acid position it is a Histidine. This could be very deleterious or it could be of no real significance. It all depends on what role the Glutamine plays in the protein. It might be at a critical bend of the structure, or at the core of a binding pocket. These may be important sites. Or glutamine may be in a dangling free portion of the protein, which does not perform any significant role. Then Glutamine or Histidine ... who cares? But nature has figured out which regions are important as the important regions are generally conserved across species. For if a mutation occurs that seriously affects the animal and it is transferred to its offspring, either the originator or the offspring has a reduced chance of survival. Evolutionary pressure reduces the odds that deleterious mutations are propagated to offspring since the originator is less likely to survive. The androgen receptor of apes, and likely Neanderthals, all have certain portions of their androgen receptors being very similar to ours.

Sometimes the DNA sequence is corrupted in a way so that it repeats itself using the same amino acid. The first part of the androgen receptor DNA gene called the N-terminal domain, are prone to have repeats of CAG or GGN (N can be either A, T, G or C) producing repeats of Glutamine (Q) or Glycine respectively. For example there may be 12 Q's in a row. Amazingly these sorts of repeats have been associated with attention deficit disorder, dominance and aggression, prostate cancer and infertility in men. This is a reminder that if you think it is irrelevant whether the amino acid sequence is ETTQKLT... or ETTQQQQQQKLT..., think again. As it turns out, we and chimpanzees, gorillas, orangutans, and gibbons all have similar repeats which adds credence to your significant other's claim that you sometimes act like a baboon.

The DNA in the nucleus is wrapped up into 23 chromosomes. The chromosome is diploid, meaning that there are two sets of DNA, one from each parent. So there are two copies of each gene. However, chromosome number 23 is a special case. It is the sex chromosome and women have an X-X pair while men have an X-Y. The Y chromosome is downright puny, being only about one third the size of the X chromosome. Men's sexual function is far less complex than women's as we do not conceive children. We just willingly help make them. The egg has only one copy, which must be X since it is from the mother, while the sperm has a 50-50 change of being either X or Y, producing girl or a boy with equal probability. The Y chromosome in men only carries 78 genes, a pittance of the total genes in the pool (~22,000). Genes that predispose men to prostate cancer occur on many chromosomes. The androgen receptor gene itself is ironically located on the X chromosome (Xq11-q12).

Cancer cells sometime form their own rules. A serious mutation is a state called aneuploidy, indicating having the wrong number of a specific chromosome. Instead of having two copies of a chromosome, there may be more, or chromosomes may be missing, apparently gone AWOL. Or it may be that there are small pieces of chromosome that exist all by themselves. More than two copies, or having extra pieces, of chromosomes can produce far more protein than is desired or needed. The androgen receptor in prostate cancer is found in some cases to be in such a gene amplification state. We go on androgen deprivation therapy and become fat, with enlarged breast and hot flashes — and our heroic attempt is defeated by this state of amplified AR production.

Even more bizarre mutations are found where parts of one chromosome may end up in the middle or end of a different chromosome. This can produce fused-proteins, a sort of two-headed monster with one head created from the genes of one protein and another head from another protein.

The body has many checks and balances to eliminate these kinds of defects — usually by signaling the cell to die, a programmed death called apoptosis. Or the immune system will target these abnormal cells and destroy them. But in cancer, there are failures that allow the cells to live on.

An important mutation that occurs in the Androgen receptor gene is a copy number variation. This means that a section of DNA is repeated more that its "wild-type" (normal) number, causing a protein to be expressed more or less that it should be. For the androgen receptor, the problem is that the gene is duplicated too many times. The caustic result is that there are too many androgen receptors produced. This leads to CRPC.

Luck And Cancer

Oh, I am fortune's fool! William Shakespeare

The primary cause of cancer is mutations in the DNA code. Recent work in 2015, and reported in the premier journal *Science,* looked at cancer of all forms with a broad brush to determine what produced the mutations.
The conclusion is that two thirds of all cancers are produced by "bad luck." The remaining ones are due to environmental effects and heredity. Luck comes in each time a cell divides. A dividing cell has to separate its two strands of DNA of the double helix and create two new strands for the daughter cell. There is a very small chance that in performing this miracle, a mistake is made. It's much like making a copying

error when one copies a letter. The cells that make the error and propagate it forward are stem cells. (More on stem cells in Chapter 7.) Like queen bees growing a colony, each stem cell may produce thousands of progeny. If an error is made in DNA replication and it is in the stem cell, it can begin producing a colony of cancerous cells that follow their own rules.

What is found in the 2015 report is that the risk of developing cancer over a lifetime in a specific tissue type increases with the total number of stem cell divisions within that tissue. This means that tissues that do not have many stem cell divisions have a low risk of cancer. Similarly those tissues that have many total stem cell divisions are more prone to cancer. For example pelvic osteosarcoma has a low lifetime risk of 0.003% and has an estimated 3 million stem cell divisions. High-risk basal cell carcinoma has a much higher risk of 30% and has about 4 trillion stem cell divisions. Looking at 31 different cancers produced a correlation between stem cell division and cancer occurrence. The analysis explains why some cell tissue is far more prone to cancer than another, and leads to the conclusion that these random, stochastic, bad-luck events are the ultimate cause of about 2/3 of all cancer occurrences. Unfortunately breast and prostate cancers were not included in the analysis, presumably because of the uncertainty in obtaining an estimate of their stem cell division numbers.

Splice Variants

Gene expression is an enormously complex phenomenon. This is made clear by the type of mutated protein called a splice variant. The goal of gene expression is to read the DNA and to transcribe it into messenger RNA (mRNA) that is then translated into protein. (The dogma of biology, DNA => mRNA => protein.) Not all of DNA is the same. DNA contains unimportant regions called introns and important regions called exons. The code is not just a continuous string of exons that directly transcribe to mRNA. It reads more like exon1-intron-exon2-intron-exon3... The introns need to be excised and the introns spliced together. If you created the universe, you might not have done it this way, but that is the way it is. The splicing may not always be the same. For example, the full-length mRNA may be composed of exon1-exon2-exon3..., while an alternate splicing may leave out exon2 producing exon1-exon3.... The alternate mRNA when translated produces a different protein. Perhaps the protein is functionally the same as the full-length protein, but it need not necessarily be so.

Alternate splicing produces many different kinds of mRNA molecules called isoforms. Each isoform has a different subset of exons. One may wonder what advantage splice variants have. The numerous possible splice variants increase the pool of proteins that are possible with a certain number of genes. This creates protein diversity – a serious amount of it. Also, splice variants are a way of regulating transcription, as they result in degradation of mRNA.

Alternate splicing is a relatively new area of research in regards to prostate cancer. The known splice variants that are important in PCa are those of the androgen receptor gene. Clinically relevant AR isoforms are AR-V7 and ARv567es. The AR-V7 (androgen receptor variant 7) is particularly important as it produces an androgen receptor that no longer needs androgen to be activated. When a long protein folds it produces clumpy regions called domains. Two important domains of the androgen receptor are the ligand binding domain, and the DNA binding domain. The AR-V7 variant is missing the androgen-binding domain on the AR protein that binds androgen. One would hope that such a malformed androgen receptor simply would be non-functional. But unfortunately it is functional. Androgen receptors are transcription factors; this means it binds to DNA and causes genes to be expressed. Quite remarkably, with the androgen-binding domain missing the androgen receptor still acts as a transcription factor but without the need of androgens. AR-V7 is in a constant state of activation and causes the cell to express proteins. This is disastrous and leads to PCa cell growth and replication. Additionally, the

AR-V7 variant causes a larger set of genes to be expressed than the full length AR, and the larger set includes those that promote adverse tumor behavior. The bottom line is that our attempts at androgen deprivation therapy and first- and second-generation antiandrogen drug therapy no longer work. Cancer finds a way to win yet again.

The Bad News of AR-V7

These results came in September 2014 from an important study headed by researchers at John Hopkins University. It studied the effect on AR-V7 on patients with CRPC taking either Enzalutamide or Abiraterone (but not both). It was a small study of 31 patients taking Enzalutamide and 31 taking Abiraterone. All had metastases.

Patients had their blood drawn and circulating tumor cells (CTCs) were searched for and collected. About 90% of patients had CTCs; only patients with CTCs found in their blood were included in the study. There are very few CTC cells in a 7.5ml blood draw test tube. It is amazing that so few (say 5) cells can be found. Antibodies are used to capture these few cells.

Once the cells are captured, a difficult biotechnology procedure is followed to determine what these cells were expressing as mRNA to be translated into ARs. These mRNA molecules were examined to determine if they were coding for full length (normal AR) or for the AR-V7 splice variant of the AR.

The analysis involves converting the mRNA back to DNA. We want DNA because of the Nobel Prize winning technique of polymerase chain reaction (PCR) that allows us to make large amounts of DNA, from tiny amounts, so that it can be analyzed. But first the RNA must be converted into DNA. The dogma of biology is DNA => RNA => Protein. We need to reverse this starting with RNA and creating DNA. An enzyme, reverse transcriptase, does this. It is a "trick" we learned from retroviruses like HIV. Retroviruses infect cells with RNA, which is converted into DNA by reverse transcriptase, and then inserted into the DNA of the host cell permanently infecting it.

Once we have large amounts of DNA, one can "run a gel" (agarose gel electrophoresis) in which DNA travels in a viscous gel (A special kind of Jell-O) under the influence of a large electric field (voltage). The distance it travels after a certain time can be correlated with its length by comparing with known length standards. Full length AR coding DNA does not travel as far down the gel as shortened AR-V7 coding DNA. So it is now easy to determine will gel electrophoresis what a patient has—full length ARs or the very undesirable AR-V7 variant.

Those that expressed AR-V7 also expressed the full length AR. Generally the full length AR was the most dominant, with the AR-V7 variant ranging from 1.8% to 50%. Those that expressed AR-V7 also tended to have more AR being expressed.

Table 6-2	Abiraterone treatment		Enzalutamide treatment	
Number total	31		31	
Number AR-V7	6		12	
	AR-V7		AR-V7	
PSA response	Yes	No	Yes	No
[+] Drop > 50%	0	17	0	10
[+] Drop 0-50%	0	5	1	6
[-] Increase 0-50%	2	1	4	2
[-] Increase >50%	4	2	7	1
	6	25	12	19

Table 6-2 shows the results of the study concerning the best PSA response each patient experienced as a percentage of their starting PSA level (baseline level). The results are quite remarkable. Of the 6 Abiraterone-treated patients with the AR-V7, none had a positive response [+] (that is a drop) in their PSA, while 22 of 25 of those with full length AR had a positive [+] response. Similarly of the 12 Enzalutamide-treated patients with AR-V7, only 1 had a

positive response, while 16 of 19 of those with AR-V7 had a positive response.

Other secondary end points of the study were PSA progression-free survival times (time before PSA increases) and overall survival. The median times for these is shown in **Table 6-3**. Again those with the AR-V7 variant did far worse than those without the variant. The trial was short and this resulted in median times not being reached for those without the AR-V7 variant (not met).

It had been known that some patients benefit from Abiraterone or Enzalutamide, while others do not. The 2014 Johns Hopkins study gives a partial answer as to why. These researchers found little or no benefit of Abiraterone or Enzalutamide for AR-V7 producing patients.

Table 6-3	Abiraterone treatment		Enzalutamide treatment	
	With AR-V7	No AR-V7	With AR-V7	No AR-V7
Median PSA progression free survival time (Months)	1.3	Not met	1.4	6
Median Overall Survival Time (Months)	10.6	Not met	5.5	Not met

This suggests a personalized medicine application— having a patient's CTCs checked for the AR-V7 variant. Those with the splice variant may not choose to undergo 2nd-generation antiandrogen therapy since there is likely (but not absolutely) to be no benefit. This saves costs, and also the side effects of these drugs. Unfortunately we are not there yet for a personalized test in a mass market. CTCs can be measured, but the mRNA-reverse transcriptase-PCR steps are time consuming. It will come.

What is needed is a strategy to not only interfere with the action of full-length androgen receptors (as does

88

Enzalutamide and Abiraterone Acetate), but interfere with
the action of AR-V7 or to block the production of AR
variants.

Blocking AR-V7

Are you a friend of Tapeworms? Probably you are
not. However, let's give them thanks for the role they have
played in the search of drugs to block AR-V7. Drugs that
attack parasites are called anti-helminthic drugs. One such
drug, Niclosamide, has been in use over 50 years and was
FDA approved in 1982. What do tapeworms and PCa cells
have in common. Nothing that I am aware of—the discovery
of Niclosamide as a PCa drug is based more on brute force
rather than a deep understanding of connections.

In 2014 a study at University of California-Davis was
"designed to identify inhibitors of AR variants and test its
ability to overcome resistance to enzalutamide." The strategy
to uncover potential useful drugs is to screen an array of
approved drugs and evaluate their effects on prostate cell
cultures. The library used is the "The Prestwick Chemical
Library®" which contains 1280 small molecule drugs that are
selected because of their diversity and low toxicity ("safe")
in humans. It is a shotgun approach, and once candidates are
found the real work starts.

The method to screen a drug is to grow cultures of
PCa cells and add the drug to the cell culture. Cultures will
grow in colonies that look like freckles in a Petri dish. One
counts colonies to get a handle on whether the drug inhibits
or eliminates growth compared to a no-drug control sample.
Being studied here is resistance to Enzalutamide due to the
AR-V7 splice variant. There are several human PCa cell
lines and two are particularly important here, CWR22Rv1
and VCaP. These cell lines express the AR-V7 splice variant
and are resistant to Enzalutamide. Another cell line explored
was C4-2, which was grown with Enzalutamide for one year
and it too became resistant to Enzalutamide. It expressed
enhanced levels of full length AR and the AR-V7 variant. At
that point it is renamed C4-2B.

One experiment will be described to illustrate the methodology. Four cell cultures were compared using several cell lines. The cultures have (Enzalutamide, Niclosamide) additions of (-,-), (+,-), (-,+) and (+,+) where – means absent and + means present (at specific concentrations of course). For example (-,+) means Enzalutamide not present and Niclosamide present. The Enzalutamide-resistant AR-V7 CWR22Rv1 and C4-2B cell lines with (-,-), (+,-), (-,+) all grew just fine. The great news is that (+,+) grew very little. It is the combination of Enzalutamide and Niclosamide that halts PCa growth—the Enzalutamide blocks the normal ARs and Niclosamide blocks or destroys the AR-V7. If both receptors are not blocked, the cells grow.

Mice were used to determine if tumor growth is affected in a living animal. CWR22Rv1 cells were injected into the flanks of mice, and tumors allowed to grow until about 50-100 mm^3 in volume. The mice were divided into four groups and treated with a (Enzalutamide, Niclosamide) as (-,-), (+,-), (-,+) and (+,+) according to group. The dosages were 25mg/kg for Enzalutamide and 25mg/kg for Niclosamide. Tumors were then measure for volume in time, and harvested after 3 weeks. The group given no drugs, (-,-), grew tumors after 3 weeks to about 900mm^3, an average from 10 mice. The Enzalutamide only group, (+,-), had tumor volumes roughly of the same size. Surprisingly, the Niclosamide only group (-,+), had average tumor volumes much smaller in comparison, about 350mm^3. The best results came from the cooperative effects of the combination therapy of Enzalutamide and Niclosamide, (+,+), which produced average tumor volumes after 3 weeks of about 150mm^3.

These mouse model results are most encouraging. Three points need to be emphasized; (i) Enzalutamide produced virtually no benefit for resistant PCa tumors, (ii) Niclosamide alone produced a benefit, and (iii) a significantly greater benefit was obtained with a combination treatment of Enzalutamide and Niclosamide. There is a final fourth point that must not be forgotten; (iv) the growth of the

90

tumors continued upon application of Enzalutamide and Niclosamide. The tumors volume did not shrink after three weeks. An optimist might hope a longer time may be needed for shrinkage to occur.

What exactly is a tapeworm drug doing to slow down the progression of PCa? The research produced several conclusions on its actions. The first is that Niclosamide degrades the AR-V7 protein. Every cell has protein sentries that search for damaged proteins and destroy them by cutting them up. The complex protein machine that does this is the proteasome. Besides degradation, Niclosamide also interferes with the transcriptional activity of AR-V7. Transcription factors are the keys that turn on genes of the cells. Reducing transcription quiets down the cell so that it is not growing or reproducing. PSA is just one gene that is expressed and this work concludes that Niclosamide reduces the transcription activity this gene also.

This research is all preclinical. Will all of it or any of it ever wind up being useful in human with Enzalutamide resistant prostate cancer is unknown. It will likely be many years before Phase I, II and III trials are completed, assuming they even start. That's the negative outlook. The positive outlook is that the drug is out there, it is generic, FDA approved for other indications, its side effects are well known, and has low toxicity. It is being studied for other cancers as well (ovarian, colorectal cancer, acute myeloid leukemia, and breast).

Mutations

In 2012 a large multi-institutional group featuring the University of Michigan, Howard Hughes Medical Institute, Compendia Bioscience, Yale, and Brown Universities performed a study of mutations and amplification of genes in prostate cancer. There are many groups doing this kind of work, as it is quite important. This group investigated a variety of aberrations — mutations, copy number gains and losses, and chromosomal fusions of two or more genes. What these researches did was to take

132 samples from 50 different prostate cancer patients that had been heavily treated for metastatic CRPC (mCRPC). Especially unique about this study is that the samples from these patients (unfortunately) were taken from autopsies. I'll call this the "Autopsy Study." The cells came from soft tissue (liver, pancreas, lung, adrenal, and others) and of course from bone. As a comparison, there were also 11 samples from the prostates (radical prostatectomy) of patients with localized but high-grade prostate cancer.

Before we get into the genetic aberrations, lets take a look at some statistics from those that succumbed to the disease from mCRPC. The study was not designed to study survival, but mutations. I'll look at survival times as I found it revealing. However, there may be confounding effects that alter the interpretation or conclusions, since this was not part of the study design; but it is revealing nonetheless. There were 50 patients but only for 47 of them do we have full data, so only those 47 are shown. We look at their survival time as a function of their PSA level at time of diagnosis. I've grouped them into 2 groups, those with "low" PSA (< 1000 ng/ml, 33 patients) and those with very high PSA (>1000 ng/ml, 14 patients). The data shows some striking features (**Figure 6-1**). First inspect the "low" PSA patients. Those with very low PSA, say between 5-200 (left quarter of Figure 6-1), have survival times that have no clear trend with PSA at diagnosis. There is a slight hint that high PSA near 800 at diagnosis leads to low survival. But the graph for very high PSA patients (>1000) contradicts this. Survival with a very high PSA at diagnosis shows again no significant trend. In fact the average survival time for the low PSA group is 98.7 months, while the high PSA group has an average survival of 99.7 months, an almost identical result. An asterisk in the two panels of **Figure 6-1** indicates the average survival time and PSA for each group.

One can try to perform numerical fitting, e.g. inverse relationship like Survival = a/(PSA+b) (a,b are constants), to try to convince yourself that a low PSA at diagnosis should extend lifetime, but this data shows no such obvious trend. All the patients in this study were heavily treated for prostate cancer—a likely potential confounding factor that may make this sample not "typical." But the highly treated group is clearly where I want to be in—anything to fight the beast.

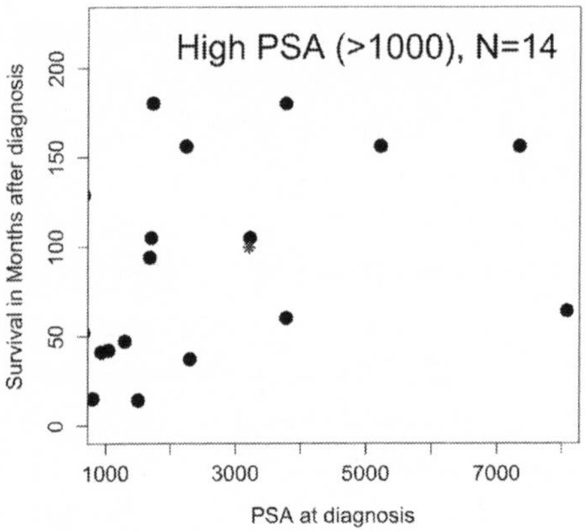

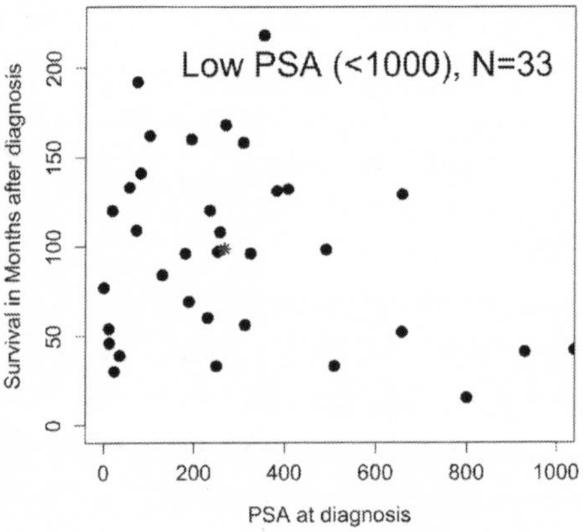

Figure 6-1. Data from Autopsy Study. Survival time after diagnosis vs. PSA level at diagnosis. The data is binned into either "low" PSA (<1000) or high PSA (>1000). An asterisk (*) shows average values in each panel. Data from CS Grasso et al., Nature 487, 239 (2012).

Now getting back to genetic alterations. The genome contains genes as well as "junk" DNA whose purpose is ill defined. But even the gene portion of the DNA is a mixture of good parts called exons and irrelevant parts called introns. A gene may contain …exon-intron-exon-intron-… and this is translated in an RNA molecule with the same basis structure. Now Enzymes come to work on the RNA cutting out the introns and splicing back together the exon parts to form the actual code for the to be translated into protein. This is called a mature RNA. The splicing is like cutting out the sections of an old 8mm movie where the bad parts with torn sprockets need to be cut out and the remaining film spliced back together. (I used to work in the St. Louis Public Library during high school and college doing work similar to this on educational films.) All this sounds impossible in a cell, but that is the way it works. The exome is the term used to describe genes where only the actual exon structure is sequenced. This is much shorter than the whole genome and of the genes themselves. It is the part we care about.

Exome-Sequencing is the sequencing of the exome of a cell. Sequencing the transcriptome is a subset of exome sequencing in that the transcriptome only sequences genes that are expressed in a specific cell. Each kind of cell is signaled to express different sections of the exome. Prostate cells express very differently than liver cells. The researchers looked at both the exome and the transcriptome, but most of the results are for the exome. Prostate cancer cells express many genes related to "maleness" that are controlled by the androgen receptor. The goal was to sequence the exome of the mCRPC prostate cells and see what aberrations exists within them. The formal goal was to study mutations. As mentioned earlier, the cells came from soft tissue and bone.

The primary aberrations that were found are shown in **Table 6-4**. There are many others, but we are reviewing the major ones to get a flavor for the troubles involved.

First some general results. Although mutations were found, the rate was fairly low, only about two per one million bases. That does not mean they are unimportant, and the androgen receptor was one that did in fact often have single point mutations. These occurred in the metastatic group only, with about 10% of the metastatic samples having a point mutation of the androgen receptor gene. These may be very important in that such a mutation could possibly cause the AR to be independent of androgen and work even without it, making androgen blockade ineffectual.

Another general result is CRPC is found to be monoclonal. This means that the tumor formed generally comes from a single renegade cell. It has a fingerprint of aberrations that are preserved as it divides, and all its successors have its same deviant properties. But at the same time prostate cancer is also heterogeneous. This monoclonal focus can produce a mutation or aberration that creates another monoclonal line. This second one may be a dud and die out or it could be far worse and be more aggressive. This is the fight we face—an on-the-move enemy that is constantly changing. If we are lucky this does not happen.

The androgen receptor (AR) is the major player in the prostate cancer story—both in localized and in advanced prostate cancer. The purpose of androgen deprivation is to derive the androgen receptor its signal to have the cancer grow. The AR communicates directly with the androgen targeted genes of the DNA and signals it to respond—one response is to grow and divide.

We discussed the AR in Chapter 3. For now suffice it to say that these experiments find that the production of the androgen receptor is amplified in half the samples with CRPC, and another 10% had point mutations. Interestingly none of the 11 high-grade untreated **localized** prostate cancer showed either mutations or amplification through copy number variations or over-expressing genes. This is certainly telling, and suggests at least one of the major differences between localized prostate cancer that largely can still be eradicated and metastatic prostate cancer on the loose and incurable.

PTEN works in an opposite way to the androgen receptor. PTEN is a tumor suppressor that helps to suppress tumors by cutting off phosphate groups, a common small chemical group that changes the actions of certain proteins. Without this protein, the cell becomes less regulated which

Table 6-4. **Genetic aberrations**	Purpose	Aberration (* discussed below.)
AR The androgen receptor	Directs DNA to express when activated by androgens.	Too many are produced and some mutated. *
PTEN Phosphatase and tensin homolog	Tumor suppressor	Too few are produced. *
TP53 Gene for Tumor Protein p53	Tumor suppressor. Guardian of the genome.	Too few produced, and mutations. *
APC Adenomatous polyposis coli	Tumor suppressor, and affects cell adhesion.	Too few are produced, and some are mutated. *
ETS2 An erythroblast transformation-specific (ETS) family member.	Transcription factor: Controls turning on/off a gene by binding to DNA.	Deleted in approximately 1/3 of mCRPC. Often caused by the TMPRSS:ERG2 fusion. *
TMPRSS:ERG2 fusion. TMPRSS2 is Transmembrane protease, serine 2. ERG2 is ETS Related Gene 2.	A common prostate cancer fusion protein, especially in CRPC. ERG2 plays a role in chromosomal translocations.	Over-expression
ZFHX3 Zinc finger homeobox 3	Tumor suppressor	Too few produced, and mutations
FOXA1	AR collaborating factor.	

leads to enhanced growth and rapid division. PTEN is under-expressed by reduced copy number in 37% of the mCRPC autopsy group. A similar reduction is found in the prostates of the prostatectomy patient group (5 out of 11). This suggests that this aberrant appears early. Mutations are also found in about another 10% in either group. PTEN is a bad actor in many different cancers besides prostate cancer. Actually, it's a good actor but, unfortunately, fails to be present for the show.

TP53 is the gene to make the tumor suppression protein p53. p53 plays many roles in regulating the cell by its action in the transcription of various regulatory genes. This protein regulates genes of other proteins for DNA repair mechanisms, and if repair is difficult, p53 helps to activate apoptosis (cell death). These are critical functions for if repairs are not made of damaged genes, the cell becomes genetically unstable and spirals into a catastrophic decline. Such cells are unable to follow instructions and become selfish searching for their own survival and not that of the body they are in. These militants would normally be tagged for programmed cell death, apoptosis, but without p53 this too becomes depressed. In 1992 it started to become clear that p53 was a primary protein in preventing cancer, and was then nicknamed "The Guardian of the Genome," as it plays a role in many different cancers. To add to the potential troubles, p53 may bind to other aberrant proteins taking it effectively out of circulation. In the mCRPC samples, about 20% were not producing enough of this gene by reduced copy numbers or deletions, and another 30% had point mutations of the gene. The prostates of the advanced but localized group showed only mutations and no copy number reductions, but recall there were only 11 such cases. p53 will come up again in Chapter 10 when we discuss Metformin. By way of information, the name p53 comes from its position when running a gel that separates proteins according to molecular weight. It lies at a position of molecular weight 53 kilodaltons. Not knowing what it was initially, its discoverers simply named it as protein 53, or p53. It's like naming a masked boxer b109, boxer of weight 109kg.

PTEN and p53 are both tumor suppressors and have a synergy between them with one cooperating with the other. PTEN is thought to police the stability of p53, while p53 acts to boost the expression of PTEN. This illustrates how events can easily cascade out of control. For if PTEN becomes deficient, p53 becomes more active and can help to counter it. That is unless p53 too fails on the job, so that the cooperative system falls apart.

APC plays two differing roles. One role is as tumor suppressor and the other affects the way cells adhere to each other. Lack of adhesion of cells can make them prone to metastases. It is found in the mCRPC group that about 10% of patients have a mutated gene and another 10% have a reduced copy number of the gene leading to too little of the protein being made. None of the 11 advanced but localized prostate cancers had mutations or reduced copy number, which reinforces the concepts that aberrations of this gene have a link, perhaps weak, with metastases. However, it's also worth noting that all of the 11 localized cancers had Gleason scores between 7 and 9. None were 10, the most aggressive form and more prone to metastasize.

The expression of genes is highly regulated. One class of regulators is "transcription factors." These are proteins that bind to DNA to signal other proteins and enzymes to form a cohort so that genes are turned on or turned off. The goal of protein expression is to transcribe the DNA into a messenger molecule, messenger RNA (mRNA) that carries the code so that it can be translated into the appropriate protein. Transcription factors are like traffic cops allowing or disallowing the transcription process. It has been estimated that 8% of all the human genome are transcription factors—that's a lot of traffic cops to maintain order. Their large numbers offer many ways in which the control system can go wrong. ETS2 is one transcription factor that is often aberrant in mCRPC. It is missing in about a third of mCRPC cases in the Autopsy Study.

98

References

Comparison of the androgen receptor CAG and GGN repeat length polymorphism in humans and apes, K-W Hong, E Hibino, O Takenaka, I Hayasaka, Y Murayam, S Ito and M Inoue-Murayama, Primates 47, 248-254 (2006).

A Structure for Deoxyribose Nucleic Acid, JD Watson and FHC Crick, Nature 171, 737-738 (1953).

Variation in cancer risk among tissues can be explained by the number of stem cell divisions, C Tomaseti and B Vogelstein, Science 347, 78 (2015).

Oncogenes and tumor suppressor genes in prostate cancer, W Issacs and T Kainu, Epidemiological Reviews 23, 36-41 (2001).

The role of mRNA splicing in prostate cancer, AV Lapuk1, SV Volik, Y Wang, CC Collins, Asian Journal of Andrology 16, 515–521 (2014).

AR-V7 and Resistance to Enzalutamide and Abiraterone in Prostate Cancer, ES Antonarakis, C Lu, H Wang, B Luber, et al., New England Journal of Medicine 371(11), 1028-1038 (2014).

Niclosamide Inhibits Androgen Receptor Variants Expression and Overcomes Enzalutamide Resistance in Castration-Resistant Prostate Cancer, C Liu, W Lou, Y Zhu, N Nadiminty, CT Schwartz, CP Evans, and AC Gao, Clinical Cancer Research 20(12), 3198-3210 (2014).

The mutational landscape of lethal castrate resistant prostate Cancer, CS Grasso, Y-M Wu, DR Robinson, X Cao, SM Dhanasekaran, AP Khan, MJ Quist, X Jing, RJ Lonigro, JC Brender, IA Asangani, B Ateeq, SY Churn, J Siddiqui, L Sam, M Anstett, R Mehta, JR Prensner, N Palanisamy, GA Ryslik, F Vandin, BJ Raphael, LP Kunju , DR Rhodes, KJ Pienta , A Chinnaiyan & SA Tomlins, Nature 487, 239 (2012).

Crucial role of p53-dependent cellular senescence in suppression of Pten-deficient tumorigenesis, Z Chen, LC Trotman, D Shaffer, H-KL, ZA Dotan, M Niki, JA Koutcher, HI Scher, T Ludwig, W Gerald, C Cordon-Cardo and PP Pandolfi, Nature 436, 725-730 (2005).

Chapter 7

Cells of trouble

I pictured myself as a virus or a cancer cell and tried to sense what it would be like.
Jonas Salk

Cells are miniature cities within our bodies. They have a downtown nuclear core center where DNA is stored, different neighborhoods in which manufacturing of cellular components takes place, energy power plants hum keeping the cell supplied with energy, and various cargo vessels shuttling components hither and yon in a crowded landscape. In this chapter we visit this very complex cell-scape with the aim of attempting to determine what goes wrong with prostate cells to make them so destructive in our lives.

Mutations within the cell's DNA are the ultimate cause of the cells transforming from healthy to cancerous. Cancer cells reproduce wildly, and worse yet, they do not undergo apoptosis (cell death). There are two main hypotheses concerning where these mutations occur to produce disease. Both have some truth. One hypothesis is a Darwinian evolution scenario in which any of the multitudes of cells gradually develop a mutation and each mutated cell, if it has a near term survival advantage, produces a new clone of potential cancer cells or full-fledged cancer cells. Environment effects speed up the process. The second scenario is much more autocratic. Here just a few cells, stem cells, call all the shots. When one of these goes bad it multiplies and multiplies and multiplies … taking over. This is the scenario that produced "bad luck" in the previous chapter.

First let's review the evolutionary model. The progression occurs in a sequence of several discrete steps. There is a population of cells and either from hereditary effects or environmental effects (e.g. diet or exposure to carcinogens) a cell develops a mutation. If the mutation has a survival advantage it reproduces clones and they develop into their own subpopulation. A clone is an exact duplicate of the original cell with the same genetic makeup, mutations and all. Regarding cancer, the advantage is not for the patient, but for the selfish survival and reproductive capabilities of the mutant. Cells are highly regulated so that they do not become selfish. However, either the microenvironment fails or the internal cell tumor suppressors fail. Random mutations occur perhaps one in a million, but there are many cells and they reproduce many times allowing a second mutation to occur. If this mutation has a survival advantage, this double mutant reproduces forming a new clonal population. The process repeats for a triple mutant, then a four-fold mutant and so on with the mutant (or cancer) possibly becoming more and more aggressive. This basic picture explains why prostate cancer takes so long to develop, and why we develop clonal foci where a tumor is all of the same genetic makeup. Yet cancer remains heterogeneous with different clones of varying aggressiveness existing simultaneously.

The second model is the stem cell model. Stem cells are cells that are capable of developing into different kinds of cells appropriate for specific tissues or organs. The process of becoming a specific kind of cell, say a luminal prostate epithelial cell, is differentiation. Every cell has the same genome (neglecting mutations and external chemical (epigenetic) changes) so in theory any cell can develop and become any kind of tissue. But signaling from the microenvironment, local neighborhood and chemical signaling queues cause tissue to be differentiated to be a particular kind of cell.

The first version of the stem cell model is that the cells in a tumor can be grossly categorized into two groups — stem cells that produce new cells and those that that do not. Stem cells are a very small minority of cells but they are the ones that actually cause the tumor to grow. The rest are reproductively passive, but take up space and nutrients and perform their function but do not reproduce. When a stem cell divides it produces two cells. One is a clone of itself, and the other cell amazingly is a differentiated (e.g. a prostate) cell. The stem cell and its prodigy have differences in the surface protein that they express and these differences are what allow researchers to identity who-is-who and sort out which cells divide and which do not.

These notions are important as killing the passive cells makes little difference. They will be replaced soon anyway. It is the minority group of cancer repopulating cells, the stem cells, which are the ones we want to target. If we can get to these, we can shrink the tumor. This first version of a stem cell model is similar to the evolutionary model, except that not all mutated cells in a tumor cause the tumor to grow—just the minority cancer repopulating cells. The "cell of origin" for the prostate cancer is a stem cell, not just any ol' prostate cell. This type of mechanism appears to act in our sister disease, breast cancer.

The second version of the stem cell model is that a stem cell does not produce a fully differentiated (i.e. prostate) cell but only a partially differentiated cell. These partially differentiated cells are called progenitor cells. A progenitor cell divides and produces a secondary differentiated cell that is closer to a fully differentiated prostate cancer cell. The process repeats until finally it develops into a full prostate cancer cell. But like the first version, these final cells do not divide further and produce growth. The growth is still in the hands of the stem cells. So again, stem cell must be our targets.

You are probably wondering why there are these various scenarios. The reason we are losing definiteness is that the answers are not clearly known. There are bits and pieces of any of these scenarios in prostate cancer and we will describe some of the findings as the story unfolds more below. It is unsatisfying not to know the exact sequence of events for such fundamental questions. This makes prostate cancer research difficult with time being wasted down blind alleys. But that is no different from the search for answers to other big scientific questions. One must make hypotheses and test them, learning as much from failure as from success.

Prostate cancer is (most often) a cancer of epithelial cells (See **Figure 7-1**). Epithelia are two dimension sheets of cells that form linings and the walls of cavities. The prostate secretes "manly" chemicals and the two dimensional nature of epithelia gives a large surface area in which to work. The sheet contains the actual epithelia layer, but below it is the basement membrane or basal layer. Below this is a structural element giving support, the stroma layer.

The five main cell types of the epithelial layer are Luminal cells, Basal cells, Neuroendocrine cells, and Intermediate cells (not shown in Fig. 7-1), with supporting

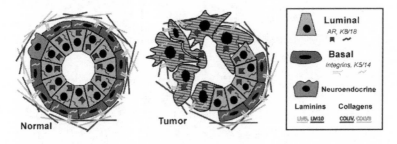

Figure 7-1. Left: The normal epithelial gland structure of the prostate showing luminal, basal and neuroendocrine cells. The stroma cells are outside the supporting structure of laminins and collagens (shown as sticks). A tumor cell in the middle panel shows a loss of basal cells and supporting structure. From SB Frank and CK Miranti, Frontiers of Oncology 3, 273, (2013).

Stroma beneath. The most numerous cells are Luminal and Basal with roughly equal numbers in the human prostate. We will discuss these different kinds of cells briefly. But our real goal is to identify which of these are causing the Trouble producing prostate cancer. Although that is a simple question, the answer is as muddy as the Missouri River, which is too thick to drink and too thin to plow.

The luminal cells are the cells that secrete man-ness into the prostate. They are androgen receptor positive (AR$^+$) meaning that they produce the AR protein and respond to androgens. Thus they produce PSA and prostatic acid phosphatase (PAP). These cells also express cytokeratins 8 and 18 (CK8, CK18). Cytokeratin proteins act as markers that can be used to determine the type of cell it is—a very useful trick for cancer diagnostics. Antibodies with light sensitive dyes are mixed with the cells and stick to a certain predetermined variety of cytokeratin. The coloring helps to identify the origin of a specific cell.

Basal cells do not express androgen receptors very highly, but they are not completely devoid of the AR. These low levels are indicated as AR$^-$ cell expression. They express CK5 and CK14, and do not express CK8 or CK18, making them distinguishable from luminal cells. They also express p63, a tumor suppressor gene very similar to p53 (Chapter 6), but the other epithelial cells do not.

Intermediate cells are rare and have properties of both a Luminal cell and a Basal cell. They express CK5 and CK14 as a Basal cell and CK8 and CK18. Note that we can identify cells if they have the following patterns of CK (5,8,14,18) expression (+,-,+,-) (-,+,-,+) and (+,+,+,+) for Basal, Luminal, and Intermediate.

Finally there are the Neuroendocrine cells. These cells are fairly rare and are not well studied. When cancerous, they are particularly difficult to treat. These cells signal nearby cells regulating them and affecting their differentiation.

Now the important questions—Which cells are the origin of prostate cancer? After prostate cancer begins, which cells are the "Cancer-repopulating cells," that is which cells progress the disease? There is a muddy area in prostate cancer research and there is no clear answer. The situation is far clearer with breast cancer where six cell subtypes have been identified. Stem cells can produce different kinds of cells by differentiation. Breast cancer is identified with six different steps in the differentiation process.

The earlier picture for the formation of prostate cancer is that the source of cancer comes from Luminal prostate cells. These cells are on the outer layer and the pathologist sees the cancer being formed in this layer and Basal cells appear absent. In 2009 a team at Columbia University and elsewhere found that Luminal cells indeed were the original source of prostate cancer, at least in studies with mice. But it was a specialized subset of Luminal prostate cells. This is fitting into the stem cell model. The subset of cells expressed a distinguishing transcription factor with the impossible name Nkx3.1. These special cells are called CAstration Resistant Nkx3.1-expressing cellS, abbreviated as CARNS. These cells could produce either normal prostate tissue or tumors. Tumors were formed when the tumor suppressor gene PTEN was deleted. Thus it appears these is a "cell of origin" of prostate cancer, perhaps of the androgen resistant variety.

Is the case closed? Not at all. Just one year later (2010) a group from UCLA found that prostate Basal cells also produce tumors, at least in mice. So there may be more that one cell of origin for prostate cancer. But what is different about Basal cells is that they do not efficiently express the androgen receptor. The UCLA researchers concluded that Basal cells may play an important role in progression after androgen withdrawal.

No one is too shocked that there are potentially two types of prostate cells that originate cancers. But there is yet another twist that was discovered in 2013, again by the UCLA group. Basal cells with certain oncogenes formed adenocarcinoma tumors with low androgen receptor levels but are transformed into Luminal-like cells. Thus basal cells that produce tumors turn into a morphed kind of Luminal cell, which is the type of cell a pathologist would normally ascribe to prostate cancer. All of this is hard to digest into a simple picture. And it is not clear if this is what actually happens in our bodies since (i) the experiments were performed on mice and (ii) specific oncogenes existed in these cells and the specific conditions may or may not occur in human subjects.

Where does this lead us? We need to know what the source of the cancer is; not just the mutations but what type of cell is the source of the cancer. It's certain that Luminal cells produce cancer, but what is not certain concerns the progression to advanced disease where androgen receptors play a lesser role. Does this condition come from Basal cells that transform into Luminal cells? We now have a weak suggestion that this may be the case. But one can see that prostate cancer and cell biology have surprises and it is unwise to conjure a mental pathway of cancer progression within cells without clear evidence.

Then there is the related question of what to do about it if we actually do know the cellular pathway. This is the translational issue of taking fundamental information about the science of the process and translating it into a therapy. Translation is around not one corner but several, so it is difficult to know how this information can yet be exploited. Our Lewis and Clark cell of origin journey has travelled only a short distance and the route ahead is getting very rocky.

References

Disruption of prostate epithelial differentiation pathways and prostate cancer development, SB Frank and CK Miranti, Frontiers of Oncology Vol 3, Article 273 (2013).

Prospective identification of tumorigenic breast cancer cells, M Al-Hajj, MS Wicha, A Benito-Hernandez, SJ Morrison, and MF Clarke, Proceedings of the National Academy of Science 100, 3983-3988 (2003).

A luminal epithelial stem cell that is a cell of origin for prostate cancer, X Wang, MK-de Julio, KD Economides, D Walker, H Yu, MV Halili, Y-P Hu, SM Price, C Abate-Shen and MM Shen, Nature 461, 495-502 (2009).

Identification of a Cell of Origin for Human Prostate Cancer, AS Goldstein, J Huang, C Guo, IP Garraway and ON Witte, Science 329, 568-571 (2010).

Prostate cancer originating in basal cells progresses to adenocarcinoma propagated by luminal-like cells, T Stoyanova, AR Cooper, JM Drake, X Liu, AJ Armstrong, KJ Pienta, H Zhang, DB Kohn, J Huang, ON Witte, and AS Goldstein, PNAS, 110 (5), 20111-20116 (2013).

Stem cells in prostate cancer: treating the root of the problem, RA Taylor, R Toivanen and GP Risbridger, Endocrine-Related Cancer 17, R273–R285 (2010).

Chapter 8

Trouble Has a Bone To Pick

Beauty may be skin deep, but ugly goes clear to the bone.
Redd Foxx

When prostate cancer spreads, it most often spreads to one of two places. One place is the immediate area around the prostate in the pelvic bed, and the other is to distant bone. Unfortunately it also finds its way to even worse places like the lung.

Here we examine when trouble finds it way to the bone, the most common site of distant metastases. Bone disease is often the cause of death in prostate cancer. The bone is of course required to support our entire bodies. Compromises in its integrity seriously affect the quality of life. Androgen deprivation therapy, which we use to treat the disease, has the additional adverse effect of advancing bone loss. ADT patients and metastatic PCa sufferers are continually worried about so-called "skeletal related events," the euphemistic medical term concerning fractures, spinal problems, and loss of mobility. We must be aware of the potential problems and how new therapies work. Additionally, the bone marrow is the source of blood cells and the cells for the immune system. These are systems vital to survival.

As we all know, the bone is a large reservoir of calcium. But it is not static. We think of bone as rock-like, but it truly is living. Bone is constantly being torn down and rebuilt. We want that reservoir of calcium to be consistently balanced, a situation referred to as homeostasis.

Our bone mass is highly regulated. There are bone-forming cells called osteoblasts (pneumonic BLast = BuiLd), and there are cells that resorb bone called osteoclasts (pneumonic CLast = CLeave). The body is filled with control systems and this is one complex example. Controlling factors include hormones, cytokines and growth

108

factors. Cancer lesions upset this mightily. **Table 8-1** introduces the main cast of players.

Table 8-1 The players	Function
Osteoblast	Bone builder -- Cells that form and build bone.
Osteoclast	Bone remover -- Cells that resorb bone.
Osteocyte	Mature bone cells.
Decoy Receptor	A receptor that binds a molecule (ligand) that keeps it from binding to its target receptor.
Receptor activator of Necrosis Factor kappaB (RANK)	An osteoclast receptor, that when activated, activates the osteoclast.
The RANK ligand (RANKL)	The molecule that binds to RANK to activate it
Osteoprotegerin (OPG)	A decoy receptor of RANKL. Removing RANKL slows down bone removing osteoclasts.

The OPG-RANK-RANKL Pathway

Homeostasis is to keep the proper amount of calcium in the bone. The OPG-RANK-RANKL pathway regulates it. Hold on—it's not so bad. Just remember the osteoclasts are removing bone and the osteoblasts are building bone. The OPG-RANK-RANKL pathway regulates them and this needs to be working properly.

The osteoclasts are large round cells that when instructed remove bone (See **Figure 8-1**). Osteoblasts are small and cubical like and build bone. These two are to work together to maintain homeostasis.

There is a receptor on the surface of osteoclasts (that remove bone) called the receptor activator of Necrosis Factor kappaB, or RANK receptor for short. What we need to know is that when it becomes activated, osteoclasts go to work and bone is removed. Too much of this and bones become weak. The signal it receives is from an activation protein RANKL. It binds to the receptor and such binding molecules are called ligands. Thus it is called the RANK ligand (RANKL). Bone cells (osteocytes) and cells in the osteoblast (builder) cell line express it. RANKL is released, binds to form a three-bound molecule (called a homotrimer). Its target is the RANK receptor. When it adheres to RANK, it activates the osteoclasts (bone resorber).

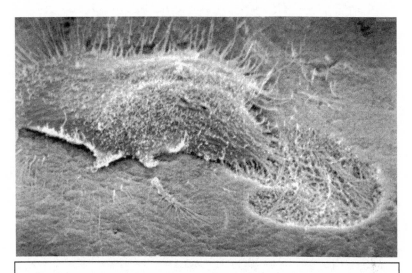

Figure 8-1. Electron microscope image of an osteoclast removing bone. Used with the kind permission from the Bone Research Society, Prof. Timothy R. Arnett.

The whole process can be modified by osteoprotegerin, hereafter called OPG. This 401 amino acid protein receptor is in the super-family of tumor necrosis factor receptors. Most tumor necrosis factor receptors are bound up on in the cell membrane. OPG is different and it is secreted. OPG was first discovered in 1997 in rats. It is expressed naturally in mice and men (and others) but its function was unknown. Mice experiments helped sort it out. A few hints go a long way. Mice expressing excess OPG exhibited increased bone density—as well as reduced osteoclast number. Fewer osteoclast leads to less bone resorption. Mice deficient in OPG developed osteopenia, reduced bone density, and an increase osteoclast activity.

From these hints you can see the origins of the OPG-RANK-RANKL pathway. Clearly OPG is controlling the removal of bone by the osteoclasts. What OPG turns out to be is a fake receptor, called a decoy receptor. When it floats around it receives the RANKL, so that RANKL never makes it to its true target the RANK receptor. This hinders the osteoclasts and slows down the removal of bone. Osteoblasts can now catch up to maintain homeostasis. The two competing reactions summarize the competition.

Reaction 1:
RANK + RANKL ==> activate osteoclast
                               (absorption of bone)

Reaction 2:
OPG + RANKL ==> 0 (harmless complex,
                              RANKL out of action)

Denosumab (Prolia, Xgeva)

Denosumab is a FDA approved drug for application in oncology to control bone loss. It is a human monoclonal (all identical) antibody that binds to RANKL. Recall that antibodies are like magnets, but stick to just one specific target. The human antibody is so specific that it does not work on rats or mice, but only primates and humans. When it binds to RANKL it is performing much the same job as OPG. It attaches to RANKL so that it does not bind to the RANK receptor, which would then activate the osteoclast to remove bone. Put another way, Denosumab is an antagonist for RANKL.

I find this story to be a very satisfying story of the practical application of science; proteins (RANK and RANKL) were discovered (1997) whose functions are unknown. We cannot discover something and not know what it does. Further experiments in mice show that they affect bone. Finally after much research the detailed pathway is uncovered. The culmination is that a "mild" intervention within the pathway can produce very positive affects. Understanding goes a long way. The company Amgen has been following this for nearly 20 years and developed Xgeva (Denosumab, Prolia). The questions of "Does it work?" and "Does it work better than Bisphosphonates?" will be re-examined after we cover Bisphosphonates, the drugs first used to delay (they say prevent) bone trouble due to metastases.

Bisphosphonates (Zoledronic Acid and More)

Tora! Tora! Tora! We are under attack. Prostate cancer mounts a silent, surprise attack on bone. It comes from multiple directions. Androgen deprivation therapy weakens bone and metastasis attacks bone. Bisphosphonates (BPs) are used to help control or slow down bone loss. Bisphosphonates are a family of chemical drugs that inhibit the resorption of bone. Resorption of bone is when osteoclasts remove bone into the blood stream weakening bone.

The general chemical structure of Bisphosphonates is shown in **Figure 8-2**. You see oxygen, phosphorus, carbon and residues (variables) R_1 and R_2. Of central importance is the P-C-P backbone consisting of two phosphorus atoms linked by a carbon atom. The two side residues R_1 and R_2 are variable, and playing with these by attaching either single atoms or other small molecules produces the range of different BPs in the family. These are acids as two –OH groups on the phosphorus release an H^+ (a proton) leaving behind O^- on the molecule.

Why do these molecules affect bone and not other body parts? Of course they do affect other body parts but they have an especially high affinity for bone. This is because bone has high amounts of calcium. Phosphates and calcium often come together and form compounds. About 70% of bone is made of the mineral hydroxyapatite $(Ca_{10}(PO_4)_6(OH)_2)$. Bisphosphonates latch onto bone by the P-C-P hook. Two oxygen atoms, one from each phosphorus, surround calcium to make the molecule stick. Variations such as changing the backbone to P-C-C-P does not seek out calcium. There is an intricate chemical balance going on concerning its affinity to calcium.

Figure 8-2. Basic chemical structure of Bisphosphonates. R_1 and R_2 are variable "residues," changing from one drug to the next. They are acids, so that the hydrogen atoms come off the —OH groups in solution, $-OH \rightarrow -O^- + H^+$.

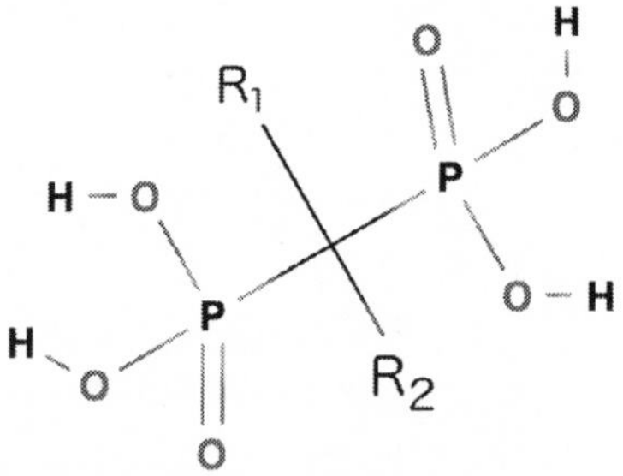

Bisphosphonates are especially attracted to sites of active bone remodeling. Starting in the blood, they are quickly cleared out and find sites of osteoclast activity on the hydroxyapatite bone surfaces.

Bisphosphonates have been known for a long time. At the same time General Lee surrendered to General Grant at Appomattox in 1865, the first BP was synthesized in Germany. They initially found use in industry to prevent build up calcium carbonate. That's the same material responsible for calcium build-up in plumbing. This provided an early clue for bone scientists—Bisphosphonates and calcium are kindred spirits. Pamidronate was approved in 1995 to reduce "skeletal related events" in multiple myeloma and breast cancer. Zoledronic acid, which is more potent, was approved for prostate cancer in 2002, also to prevent skeletal related events. Also, the ability of PBs to adhere to bone is taken advantage of in whole-body bone scintigraphy, also known as a bone scan. The radioactive element Technetium (^{99}Tc) is connected to a Bisphosphonate to image bone lesions from the γ-radiation of Technetium.

Finding bone, especially where there is bone activity, is only half the battle. The BP has to perform some beneficial function. What BPs do is enhance apoptosis (death) of osteoclast cells (cells which tear down bone) or to inhibit osteoclast attachment to bone. The mechanism of action depends on the specific BP. The mechanism of activity falls into two categories depending on whether the BP has Nitrogen in the R_2 site or not.

Table 8-2 shows a list of Bisphosphonates, their R_2 N-content, and relative potency. Those with nitrogen in the R_2 residue are more potent than those that do not. But, they are also more prone to produce osteonecrosis of the jaw (later in this chapter), death of jaw bone.

Table 8-2: Bisphophonates	N on R_2	Relative potency (After Gutta et al., 2007)
Etidronate (Didronel)	No	× 1
Clodronate	No	× 10
Tiludronate	No	× 10
Pamidronate (Aredio)	Yes	× 100
Alendronate (Fosamax)	Yes	× 1000
Risedronate (Actonel)	Yes	× 5000
Ibandronate	Yes	× 5000
Zoledronic acid (Zometa, Reclast)	Yes	× 10,000

The Non-N-BPs enter the interior of osteoclast cells and produce a cytotoxic mimic of ATP (adenosine triphosphate). This completely messes up the metabolism of the cell and results in apoptosis. It is the energy molecule that supplies energy to cells throughout the body releasing its energy when a phosphate group is cleaved off to produce ADP (adenosine diphosphate), ATP => ADP + Phosphate. The important point here is that P-C-P backbone (where P is decorated with oxygen, just as in ATP) is chemically similar to the end of ATP molecule.

Bisphosphonate is metabolized in the osteoclast cell, pairing up with ADP to produce P-C-P-O-P-5sugar-adenine. The 5sugar is a 5-ring sugar molecule and adenine happens to be the same "A" molecule as in the DNA A-T-G-C genetic code. The three molecules, ATP, ADP, and Metabolized-BP are shown schematically in the box.

ATP:	P-O-P-O-P-5sugar-adenine
ADP:	P-O-P-5sugar-adenine
Metabolized-BP:	P-C-P-O-P-5sugar-adenine

Biology is smart but not that smart. The metabolized BP molecule is mistaken for ATP. It binds to enzymes and other machinery within the osteoclast and takes the place of ATP. The problem (for the osteoclast) is that the carbon-phosphorus bond is much stronger that the oxygen-phosphorus bond. So when cleavage is attempted to change ATP to ADP and release the energy in hydrolysis, it cannot be done. The cell's energy source has dried up—its gas tank has been emptied. Osteoclast activity is shut down and bone is not removed.

The BPs with Nitrogen within R_2 behave differently. The N-BPs interrupt an important pathway that synthesizes several biomolecules necessary for proper functioning of the cell. This pathway is called the mevalonate pathway. Pathways involve a long cascade of biochemical reactions, and are modulated and enacted by enzymes. If a drug interferes with an enzyme in this pathway, it stops the dominoes from falling along the cascade. Potentially, many downstream biomolecules are no longer made. The specific enzyme that is affected by N-BPs is called the farnesyl diphosphate synthase (FPPS). It is a protein molecular machine.

In 2006 an international team studied the interaction of risedronate and zoledronate with the FPPS enzyme. This was done with x-ray crystallography. In x-ray crystallography one must first crystallize the sample, which means having many enzyme-BP complexes frozen into a crystalline lattice. X-ray crystallography does not directly make an image but produces a series of x-ray spots from which one works backwards to arrive at a structure. What is found is that the N-BP is positioned in a ligand-binding pocket within the enzyme. This is reminiscent of the binding of androgen within the androgen receptor, or RANKL binding to RANK. An important consequence of the binding of the BP within the FPPS enzyme is that there is a change in structure of the enzyme when this occurs. Changing form changes function. This disrupts the chemical mevalonate pathway, which then alters the action of the osteoclast cells.

Bisphosphonates—Do They Work?

A Phase 3 trial by an international team was reported in 2002 for the Bisphosphonate drug zoledronic acid. It specifically investigated metastatic castrate resistant prostate cancer patients (bone metastases) and to test if bone destruction and skeletal complications are reduced with Zoledronic acid (ZOL). Patients were enrolled from June 1998 through January 2001. The study was designed to proceed over 15 months with patients receiving intravenous treatment every 3 weeks. Patients were randomly assigned to one of three groups. One group received 4mg ZOL, a second group received 8mg ZOL, which was later reduced to 4mg, and one group received a placebo. The reason that the 8/4mg group had their dosage reduced is that the 8mg dosage was found to be toxic to kidneys and the dosage was reduced in June 2000. All patients received daily supplements of 500mg of calcium and 400-500 IU of vitamin D.

Table 8-3 shows the median time to first "skeletal related event" (SRE). The median time (that is when 50% of patients had an SRE) was not reached over the 420 days of the trial. An extrapolation of the data gives an estimate of about 525 days. The important point is that this time is considerably longer than both the placebo group and the 8/4mg group. A skeletal related event includes a bone fracture, bone surgery, spinal cord compression, radiation administered to the bone, or a change in cancer therapy to treat bone pain. The percentage of patients who experienced SREs is smallest in the 4mg Zoledronic acid group and largest for the placebo group.

Table 8-3	Number	Median time to first skeletal related event (Days).	% with skeletal related events
Zoledronic acid (4mg)	214	Not reached (>420) (Extrapolate ~ 525)	33.2%
Zoledronic acid (8/4mg)	221	363	38.5%
Placebo	208	321	44.2%

A curious feature of the trial is that only about a third of the patients completed the 15-month trial. The researches attribute this to the short median time to progression of disease (84 days) and a short median survival time (just 15 months in the placebo group).

There is benefit demonstrated, but the demonstration is not the difference between night and day. As with most therapeutic treatments of PCa, it is not obstacle removal that occurs but rather modest obstacle reduction. What we really care about is life extension and quality of life. The study gives a grim summary that tumor progression is not changed by zoledronic acid compared to a placebo.

Denosumab—Does it work?

The FDA approved Denosumab (Xgeva) in November 2010 for prevention of skeletal-related events in patients with bone metastases from solid tumors. This includes metastatic castrate resistant prostate cancer.

Approval was based on a head-to-head Phase 3 clinical trial (NCT0031620) that compared Denosumab with

Zoledronic acid in their the ability to prevent skeletal-related events. The results of the study were published in the British Journal *Lancet* in 2011. The patients had mCRPC and had not received previous treatment with Bisphosphonates. The study was conducted between May 2006 and October 2009. Patients were randomly placed into one of two groups. One group received 120mg of Denosumab via subcutaneous injection every 4 weeks. The second group received 4mg Zoledronic acid intravenously every 4 weeks. To keep the trial blinded, the Denosumab group received an additional intravenous placebo, and the Zoledronic acid group an additional subcutaneous injection of a placebo, which masked which group each patient was in.

The results of the study are shown **Table 8-4**. There were a total number of 1,901 patients divided equally (950 vs. 951) between the two groups. The primary endpoint was the time to a patient's first skeletal related event (SRE). A skeletal related event was defined as a fracture, radiation administered to bone, spinal cord compression, or surgery to the bone. Table 8-4 shows that Denosumab was superior in preventing a first SRE compared to Zoledronic acid, and added an extra 3.6 months median time to 1st SRE (20.7 mo vs. 17.1 mo). This translates to a "Hazard ratio" of 0.82. Denosumab appears to be superior in all entries except osteonecrosis (ONJ) of the jaw, a serious side effect.

Although Denosumab appears superior, it is not hands-down superior. Other considerations like cost, adverse effects, IV vs. subcutaneous injection, and concern of ONJ will come into play. Looking at the big picture, disease progression (not including SREs) and overall survival were not significantly different between the two groups.

Denosumab and Zoledronic acid are not miracle drugs. About 40% (36-41%) of patients had an SRE during the study; this is far from eliminating such events. The most common skeletal related event was bone fracture, which occurred in 19% of Denosumab patients and 21% of Zoledronic acid patients.

Table 8-4	Denosumab	Zoledronic Acid
Number of patients	950	951
Number that experience a first skeletal related events (SRE)	341 (36%)	386 (41%)
Median time on study to first SRE	20.7mo	17.1mo
1st SRE = Fracture	177 (19%)	203 (21%)
1st SRE = Radiation to bone	137 (14%)	143 (15%)
1st SRE = Spinal cord compression	26 (3%)	36 (4%)
1st SRE = Surgery to bone	1 (<1%)	4 (<1%)
Total number of SREs. (A single patient may experience multiple events.)	494	584
Number of patients experiencing osteonecrosis of the jaw	22 (2.3%)	12 (1.3%)

Big Trouble In The Jaw—Osteonecrosis Of The Jaw

There is a risk of osteonecrosis of the jaw (ONJ) in prostate cancer patients taking Bisphosphonates or Denosumab. ONJ is a form of "bone-death" and the chance of this occurring is not slim enough to ignore—estimates are between 1 and 15%. That is a wide range due to it not being fully understood. If ONJ were a minor or moderate side effect these relatively small odds might not be a concern. But ONJ is a big-time side effect that no one would want to get. Dental work while taking these drugs tends to help bring on ONJ, so standard advice to all is to have dental issues fixed before taking these drugs. And add to that good oral hygiene. I am taking Denosumab and these issues are of great concern to me personally. The disease is already bad enough; no additional trouble is welcome from a preventative medication.

Let's first discuss Bisphosphonates. Jawbone is a bone that has a rapid turnover, and this probably is what makes it susceptible. Additionally, Bisphosphonates stay in jawbone a long time; apparently a really long time. The risk of ONJ increases with the number of infusions and dental work. It is hard to avoid serious dental work like tooth extractions for too long, but at least anticipated dental work can be taken care of before going on Bisphosphonates.

There are many confounding factors that change the risk of ONJ from Bisphosphonates.

The largest study of ONJ in Bisphosphonates in PCa patients was reported in 2014 by Brazilian urologists. The study started in 2001 and followed 318 patients for a median time of about 4.5 years. They compared patients taking Zoledronic acid ($C_5H_{10}N_2O_7P_2$) with those taking clodronic acid ($CH_4Cl_2O_6P_2$). Zoledronic acid contains Nitrogen (N) while Clodronic acid does not. Keep in mind that Zoledronic acid is about 1000 time more potent that Clodronic acid. From their study they conclude ONJ is related to the N-Bisphosphonates. This conclusion may be true, and it probably is, but their data does not clearly show this. They offer the advice that those at risk of ONJ may want to avoid switching Bisphosphonates.

The situation is quite perplexing. Let's look at what their data show (**Table 8.5**). There were four groups of PCa patients; those that took Clodronic acid, those that took Zoledronic acid, a crossover group that started with Clodronic acid and switched to Zoledronic acid and a control group who took nothing. The first three rows of the chart show the raw data. We discuss the 4th row later (the Probability row). Just two (2) of the 318 patients experienced ONJ, and the 2 patients were all crossover patience who started on Clodronic (non-nitrogen) and switched to Zoledronic (nitrogen containing). The raw data certainly suggests switching from a non-N Bisphosphonate to a N-containing one enhances the occurrence of ONJ. But this is such a special case. Many patients not in this study have gotten ONJ that were on just one drug. So the authors of this work attribute the occurrence of ONJ to the Nitrogen containing drug Zoledronic acid. If we go along with this

Table 8-5	Control	Monthly Clodronate	Zoledronic acid	Crossover: Clodronate changed to Zoledronic
Number (n)	54	156	94	14
ONJ incidence	0	0	0	2
Probability of ONJ with p=2/108=1.85%			P(0)=17.3% P(1)=30.6% P(2)=26.9%	P(0) = 77.0% P(1) = 20.3% P(2) = 2.5%

assumption, we can compute the Probability of having k incidences, P(k), in the Zoledronic and in the crossover groups. Some simple analysis shows $P(0)=(1-p)^n$, $P(1)=np(1-p)^{n-1}$, $P(2)= 1/2\ n(n-1)p^2(1-p)^{n-2}$ where n is the number in the sample and p is the probability that any one patient in that group experience ONJ. I will accept the notion, for this analysis, that it is the N-containing drugs that produce ONJ. Then an estimate of p comes from the number of ONJ incidence (2) divided by the total number of patients that took the N-containing drug (Zoledronic + Crossover group, 94+14=108). Thus p is 2/108=0.0185, or slightly less than 2%. The questioning comes in when we ask "what is the chance that these two ONJ sufferers would only be in the crossover group?" We see that the chance of two ONJ cases in the crossover group is 2.5%, and the chance of 0 ONJ cases in the Zoledronic group is 17.3%. It is the result of the crossover group that appears so unlikely; there is a 97.3% chance that either zero or 1 patient would experience ONJ. Of course these are only statistics and only indicate what is likely to happen. Picking an ace of spades from a deck of cards is also unlikely, but it happens. The results reported in the Brazilian study are either the result of a very unlucky sampling of patients or there are important uncovered effects at work.

It is noteworthy that the two patients that experienced ONJ did have dental extractions. Likely many other patients did as well. It appears wise to avoid serious dental work if possible.

Science is about data. The analysis above was concerning just the raw data of that study. But there are other measurements and data to consider. A literature review of the connection between Bisphosphonates and ONJ was reported in 2006. It reviewed 32 scientific references and the data included 225 individual patients who experienced ONJ. These were not specifically PCa patients. In fact only 7 were PCa patients, but 94% had some form of a cancer. The most frequent cancers were multiple myeloma (97 patients) and breast cancer (89 patients). Seventy-five percent (75%) were receiving chemotherapy.

The patients included in this study had developed ONJ after taking a Bisphosphonate. The median time having taken BP at diagnosis of ONJ was about 30 months. Additionally, there is one striking fact that emerged from the review. Of all the ONJ cases dug up, every single one of them had taken nitrogen-containing Bisphosphonate. The majority had taken either Pamidronate or Zoledronic acid. What we do not know is if this is a coincidence or there was some other factor. The study was seeking a Bisphosphonate-ONJ connection, and not on comparing non-N-BPs with N-BP. The 2006 review included papers from 2003-2005. Before 2003, cases were not often reported since the Bisphosphonate-ONJ connection was not realized.

The bottom line concerning ONJ and Bisphosphonates (as hazy as it is) appears to be (1) get dental work done before taking Bisphosphonates and maintain good oral hygiene, (2) don't switch from non-N to N-containing Bisphosphonates, and (3) consider using non-N-containing Bisphosphonate if ONJ is a risk or concern for you, but realize they are far less potent. Clearly, consult your oncologist and your dentist concerning these issues.

The ONJ problem does not go away using the antibody Denosumab. Denosumab seems to cause some of the same ONJ problems as Bisphosphonates, even though they are completely different drugs. I find this surprising. It was not realized that there might be a link between Denosumab and ONJ until 2010 when the first cases were reported. To get a handle on this there have been at least two retrospective analyses of clinical trials involving Denosumab where the occurrence of ONJ was analyzed. The first analysis in 2011 looked at two clinical trials A and B, which compared Denosumab head to head with Zoledronic Acid. Trial A (NCT00321464) was on breast cancer patients and Trial B (NCT00330759) on advanced cancer or myeloma (excluding breast or prostate cancers). **Table 8-6** shows the results. Both Denosumab and Zoledronic acid produce a 1-2% occurrence of osteonecrosis of the jaw.

Table 8-6 After Kyrgidis et al. 2011		
	Denosumab	
Trial	n(ONJ)/n(Patients)	% ONJ
A	20/1026	1.95%
B	10/888	1.13%
Total	30/1914	1.57%
	Zoledronic Acid	
Trial	n(ONJ)/n(Patients)	% ONJ
A	14/1020	1.37
B	11/888	1.24
Total	25/1908	1.31

The second report in 2014 retrospectively analyzed 7 clinical trials. Those results are shown in **Table 8-7**. They too show a 1-2% occurrence of ONJ in Denosumab or Bisphosphonate usage. There is a higher percentage occurrence of ONJ from Denosumab than Bisphosphonates. Because it is retrospective and a mixture of 7 different clinical trials, there are variables that are uncontrolled. For example dosages, schedule of dosage, period of administration, type of cancer and so on were different. In spite of these difficulties they give us some idea of ONJ occurrence.

Table 8-7 (after Qi et al., 2014)	
Denosumab	
n(ONJ)/n(Patients)	% ONJ
85/4585	1.85%
Bisphosphonates	
n(ONJ)/n(Patients)	% ONJ
33/2928	1.13%
Placebo	
n(ONJ)/n(Patients)	% ONJ
0/1450	0%

Many of the patients in this analysis (Qi et al.) were prostate cancer patients. A separate analysis of these patients taking Denosumab reveals an n(ONJ)/n(Patients) ratio of 55/2393. This gives a 2.30% probability of getting ONJ from Denosumab, which is slightly higher in PCa than in the amalgam of all cancers. However, the follow-up period for PCa was significantly longer for the PCa patients than in general. This is a reasonable explanation for this increase. It may not necessarily mean that prostate cancer is more prone to ONJ than other cancers. We must keep in mind that the length of time on Denosumab and its dose may be important factors in ONJ occurrence.

Radium 223 Dichloride (Xofigo)

Now we move on to radiating the lesions in the bone to stop bone loss, reduce pain, and reduce the tumor burden. We will start with a bit of chemistry and physics, which will go a long way in understanding how they work.

Bone is being remodeled constantly and cancer lesions accelerate the process. The biomineral that is predominant in bone is hydroxyapatite, with chemical composition $Ca_{10}(PO_4)_6(OH)_2$. One can see it is composed of phosphate groups PO_4, a common group in many biomolecules, the hydroxyl group OH, a fragment from splitting water, and a good amount of Calcium. Remodeling bone requires needed calcium in the region. But calcium builds bone and does not attack lesions; we need something that will attack.

Let's take a look at the first two columns of the periodic table and see what chemistry might help. Just in case you forgot, the symbols stand for the elements –Column I: Hydrogen, Lithium, Sodium, Potassium, Rubidium, Cesium, Francium; Column II: Beryllium, Magnesium, Calcium, Strontium, Barium, and Radium.

I	II
$_1$H	
$_3$Li	$_4$Be
$_{11}$Na	$_{12}$Mg
$_{19}$K	$_{20}$**Ca**
$_{37}$Rb	$_{38}$Sr
$_{55}$Cs	$_{56}$Ba
$_{87}$Fr	$_{88}$**Ra**

The column we care about is column II; this is the column with calcium. The subscripts, like 20 in $_{20}$Ca, tell us the number of protons in the nucleus, that is the total charge of the atom. Of course this positive charge attracts 20 outer negatively charged electrons, so it is overall neutral in the body. The important concept about the periodic table is that atoms in a specific column, say column II, have a similar outer arrangement of electrons—thus they behave in a similar manner chemically. For column II, there are two outer electrons that bind to other atoms and perform most of the chemistry. So 18 of the 20 electrons on calcium are not chemically effective. But all the column II elements have 2 outer electrons and can substitute for each other, at least often then can. Beryllium is toxic and Mg is metallic. So candidates that can substitute for Calcium are Strontium, Barium and Radium. The point is that the body will likely take up these three elements in bone as it does calcium. This could be problematic, as similar is not identical. However, we don't have much, if any, Sr, Ba or Ra floating around in our bodies, so the problem does not come up.

What we want is a calcium replacement that will be absorbed like calcium but kills what's nearby, our tumor lesion. Since the topic here is Radium 223, let's get to

Radium. The nucleus of atoms contains protons and neutrons. Protons are positively charged and neutrons are neutral. Elements with a small positively charged nucleus (few protons) tend to have a nucleus with about an equal number of protons as neutrons. But neutron count number can vary; these are isotopes of the same element. For example, three natural isotopes of magnesium are ^{24}Mg, ^{25}Mg, and ^{26}Mg. They all have 12 protons (or else it would not be Mg), but the isotopes have 12, 13, or 14 neutrons, similar to the proton number. The superscript (24, 25, or 26) is the atomic mass, which adds up both neutrons and protons.

Heavy elements like Ra and Fr are different. The protons in the nucleus repel each other and the nucleus is becoming less stable. The neutrons are there to dilute the protons and add extra attractive forces to hold it together. The isotope Ra 223 is ^{223}Ra, 88 protons and 223-88= 135 neutrons. This isotope has a large excess of neutrons, but just not quite excessive enough and is unstable, meaning it is radioactive. It decays (explodes) by spitting out two protons and two neutrons bound together. This is a helium nucleus, ^{4}He but we don't call it a helium nucleus because it is ejected at very high speed without its negative charge compensating electrons. It is a destructive missile called an α (alpha) particle. As we will see, that's terrific; it is an alpha emitter. In reactions there are three main types of radiation for tumor destruction; α, β (beta), and γ (gamma). β-decay is very common and it refers to high energy electrons. Electrons are very light (about 1/8000 the mass of an α particle), and they go deep into tissue. γ-Radiation is high-energy electromagnetic radiation, like an X-ray. They go deep as well. Going deep means it causes damage to much tissue, not to just the nearby tumor.

The fast moving α particles do damage like a bowling ball. They are destructive but do not go far. The important fact is that ^{223}Ra α penetration is around or even less than 100μm (micrometers), that is 0.1mm. In tissue terms, this is about the diameter of 5 cells. So it will only kill cells in its immediate surroundings. To emphasize the point further, we all know γ-rays go through the body (that's how x-rays "see" your bones), but α particles won't even go through a sheet of paper.

We do not want radioactivity around forever. ^{223}Ra has a half-life of 11.43 days. So in about 11 days we have half of what we started with, in 22 days one fourth, and in about a month one eight. In a couple of months we are down to 1/64'th of the original amount. Of course, this half-life discussion refers to the decay of Radium not excreted naturally in urine and feces. In fact, most (76%) is excreted after 7 days. The majority is excreted in feces; so regular bowel movements remove it more effectively. So Ra223 does its job, and goes away fairly quickly. For that portion no excreted, where does it go? The reaction cascade is Ra decays to Rn (Radon). That is the slow step. Other steps involving further decay are rapid and involve Rn finally ending in ^{207}Pb (lead), which is stable.

Let's review why we use ^{223}Ra. (1) Radium substitutes for Calcium because it is in the same column of the periodic table with two valence electrons, (2) ^{223}Ra is an α-emitter which keeps the damage local and does not affect distant organs (as long as it does not actually reside in these distant organs), and (3) it reduces its potency quickly to ½ its initial potency in 11 days.

There are other elements that will go to bone and emit. Two older ones are ^{89}Sr (Strontium) and ^{153}Sm (Samarium). These are both β-emitters. Strontium fits our simple picture of Column II of the periodic table; with Sr substituting for Ca. Sm is a rare-earth element that does not fit the Column II picture. β particles are not stopped nearly as quickly as α particles. For example β particles from Sr travel about 0.8cm, which is about 1/3 of an inch—a large distance compared with the size of cells.

The FDA approved Ra 223 for treatment of metastatic castrate resistant prostate cancer when there is no known visceral (internal organ) metastatic disease. The trade name is Xofigo, but was previously called Alpharadin. The clinical trial establishing its usefulness was the Alpharadin

Symptomatic Prostate Cancer trial, or the ALSYMPCA trial and was led by scientists in the United Kingdom. Besides reducing skeletal related events, bone pain and an increase in quality of life, it also showed an overall survival (OS) benefit. It is not a cure, but helps control pain and improves quality of life. Other bone therapies help relieve pain and delay skeletal related events, but Ra 223 has been shown to extend overall survival. It produced only a modest OS increase, but at least it was there. Let's look at the trial and its benefits more closely.

The ALSYMPCA trial was a double blind study of 921 men, with the randomly selected control group receiving a placebo in a 2:1 ratio (2 Ra patients to 1 placebo patient). The patients were a well-mixed group, with the only limitation being that none had visceral disease. Chemotherapy (Docetaxel) was not a factor. Some had taken it, some not, some too sick to take it. A one-month recovery from chemo was required. The patients were recruited from June 2008 to February 2011. Since then Enzalutamide, Abiraterone and Cabazitaxel have come on the scene to further enhance overall survival.

The procedure was to inject the radium solution six times separated by one-month intervals. The dose was 50kBq per kg of body mass. The Becquerel (Bq) unit means that there is one radioactive decay per second. So 50kBq is 50,000 radioactive decays per second. The primary end point was overall survival, and secondary endpoints were time to skeletal-related events or other progression indicators. During the trial, but after 528 deaths had occurred, the placebo patients were switched to Ra as it was deemed superior to the placebo. Besides the radium treatment, the patients received other best standard of care treatments for their case.

The Figure **8-3** shows the Overall Survival of the ALSYMPCA trial. What one usually looks for in overall survival are the median overall survival times, which is when half the patients have died, and half survived (glass half empty or half full). The ^{223}Ra group had median overall survival of 14.9 months while the placebo group 11.3 months. That's 3.6 months difference. It helps, every little bit helps, but it is nothing resembling a miracle cure. We want to see comparisons using years, not months. But it improves quality of life. The median time to the first symptomatic skeletal event is 15.6 month for the Ra group and 9.8 for the placebo group. Life is better for the radium group.

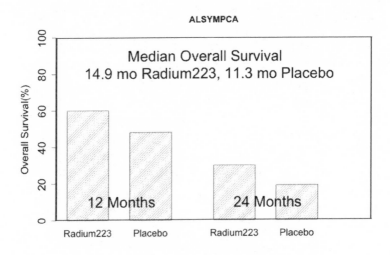

Figure 8-3. Results of Overall Survival from the ALSYMPCA trial comparing a placebo with Radium 223. Mean overall survival is increased in the Ra223 arm. (Data from C Parker et al., New England Journal of Medicine 369, 213-223 (2013).

There seem to be no additional adverse affects due to the [223]Ra treatment. Expect to be even more tired, and perhaps diarrhea. There were no clinically meaningful differences in serious adverse events between the placebo group and the [223]Ra group.

I am participating (Initiated June 2015) in NCT02023697, "Standard Dose Versus High Dose and Versus Extended Standard Dose Radium-223 Dichloride in

Castration-resistant Prostate Cancer Metastatic to the Bone."
It is a phase 2 trial by Bayer to test different dosages.

References:

Bench to bedside: elucidation of the OPG-RANK-RANKL pathway and
the development of denosumab, Nature Reviews Drug Discovery 11,
401- 419 (2012).

(Review article) Mechanisms of Bone Metastasis, GD Roodman, New
England Journal of Medicine 350, 1655-1664 (2004).

Osteoprotegerin: a novel secreted protein involved in the regulation of
bone density, WS Simonet *et al.*, *Cell* **89**, 309–319 (1997).

Bisphosphonates and osteonecrosis of the jaws: Science and rationale, R
Gutta and PJ Louis, Oral surgery, oral medicine, oral pathology, oral
radiology, and endodontology 104(2), 186-193 (2007).

Safety of I.V. Nonnitrogen Bisphosphonates on the Occurrence of
Osteonecrosis of the Jaw: Long-Term Follow-Up on Prostate Cancer
Patients, P Rodrigues, F Hering, and
M Imperio, Clinical Genitourinary Cancer, in Press: Available online 23
October (2014).

Bisphosphonates and osteonecrosis of the jaw: cause and effect or a post
hoc fallacy?, T. Van den Wyngaert, MT Huizing and JB Vermorken,
Annals of Oncology 17, 1197-1204 (2006).

The molecular mechanism of nitrogen-containing bisphosphonates as
antiosteoporosis drugs, KL Kavanagh, K Guo, JE Dunford, X Wu, S
Knapp, FH Ebetino, MJ Rogers, RGG Russell, and U Oppermann,
Proceedings of the National Academy of Science 103(20), 7829–7834
(2006).

A Randomized, Placebo-Controlled Trial of Zoledronic Acid in Patients
With Hormone-Refractory Metastatic Prostate Carcinoma, F Saad, DM
Gleason, R Murray, S Tchekmedyian, P Venner, L Lacombe, JL Chin, JJ
Vinholes, JA Goas, and B Chen, Journal of the National Cancer Institute
94(19), 1458-1468 (2002).

Denosumab versus zoledronic acid for treatment of bone metastases in
men with castration-resistant prostate cancer: a randomised, double-blind
study, K Fizazi, M Carducci, M Smith, R Damião, J Brown, L Karsh, P

Milecki, N Shore, M Rader, H Wang, Q Jiang, S Tadros, R Dansey, and C Goessl, Lancet 377(9768), 813–822 (2011).

Denosumab-related osteonecrosis of the jaws, A Kyrgidis and KA Toulis, Osteoporosis International 22(1), 369–370 (2011).

Risk of osteonecrosis of the jaw in cancer patients receiving denosumab: a meta-analysis of seven randomized controlled trials, W-X Qi, L-N Tang, A-N He, Y Yao and Z Shen, International Journal of Clinical Oncology 19, 403–410 (2014).

Alpha Emitter Radium-223 and Survival in Metastatic Prostate Cancer, C. Parker, S. Nilsson, D. Heinrich, S.I. Helle, J.M. O'Sullivan, S.D. Fosså, A. Chodacki, P. Wiechno, J. Logue, M. Seke, A. Widmark, D.C. Johannessen, P. Hoskin, D. Bottomley, N.D. James, A. Solberg, I. Syndikus, J. Kliment, S. Wedel, S. Boehmer, M. Dall'Oglio, L. Franzén, R. Coleman, N.J. Vogelzang, C.G. O'Bryan-Tear, K. Staudacher, J. Garcia-Vargas, M. Shan, Ø.S. Bruland, and O. Sartor for the ALSYMPCA Investigators, New England Journal of Medicine 369, 213-223 (2013).

Chapter 9

Toxins For Trouble: Chemotherapy

What does not kill me makes me stronger. Friedrich
Nietzsche.

Taxanes are chemotherapeutic drugs for cancer. This
chapter will explore how they act in prostate cancer. The
most familiar of the taxane family of drugs is Docetaxel.
Docetaxel (Taxotere) is the first line chemotherapy drug for
prostate cancer. Using Docetaxel means you are into the big
guns fighting cancer. It is a frightful experience as
chemotherapy has so many side effects. It's a crapshoot as to
whether you experience serious ones or not. Docetaxel was
FDA approved for metastatic castrate resistant prostate
cancer on May 19, 2004. Just three months later, on August
18, 2004, approval was similarly given for breast cancer.
However, taxanes have a much longer history in treatment of
cancer in general. Nearly 25 years ago (1992) the FDA
approved the related taxane drug Taxol for metastatic
ovarian cancer. Today many cancers are treated with taxanes.
Table 9.1 lists the major players in this chapter.

Docetaxel is member of the taxane family of drugs.
First was Paclitaxel (Taxol), but Docetaxel largely replaces it
due to Docetaxel's more potent effects. Taxanes work in a
unique manner—interrupting cell division from one mother
cell into two daughter cells. The interference leads to cell
death. It does this by changing the properties of microtubules
as will be discussed below. This is serious business since cell
division is a natural process that cells in your body undergo.
Cancer cells divide rapidly, and that is being relied on so that
not every cell in your body is destroyed. Rapidly dividing
cells are more likely to be affected by Docetaxel than an
average cell. But other rapidly dividing cells are also
strongly affected like hair and nails. So your hair falls out

132

and fingernails turn black, or grow irregularly, or simply fall off. But these are the "not serious" side effects.

Table 9-1. **Major chemo drugs**	
Taxane	A generic name for a class of anticancer chemotherapy agents.
Docetaxel (Taxotere)	A first line chemotherapy drug for prostate cancer. Acts on microtubules during cell division.
Paclitaxel (Taxol)	The first taxane to be discovered.
Mitoxantrone (Novantrone)	An early chemotherapy drug (not a taxane). Acts on DNA topoisomerase during cell division.
Cabazitaxel (Jevtana)	A second line chemotherapy taxane drug for prostate cancer. Used to counteract Docetaxel drug resistance. Acts to prevent chemo drug removal from the cell.
Cisplatin	A platinum-based drug used for aggressive prostate cancer variants. Glues-up DNA to trigger cell death.
Etoposide	A drug sometimes used with Cisplatin that acts on DNA topoisomerase during cell division.

Docetaxel is a relatively large organic molecule of 111 atoms of chemical formula $C_{43}H_{53}NO_{14}$. However it has a complex shape. Its predecessor, Paclitaxel, was obtained initially not from a laboratory, but naturally from the bark of the scarce Pacific yew plant. Its discovery is one of those events that remind us to treasure and preserve the diversity of plants on earth. Testing chemicals from thousands of plants for anti-cancer properties led to its discovery. Nature has done most of the hard work in creating the complex shape and composition of this molecule. Since the plant source is rare, chemists took it from there, and used a similar molecule from the European yew and modified it slightly to reproduce Paclitaxel. The European yew tree (*Taxus baccata*) is far more common than its Pacific cousin, and is a poisonous plant because it produces taxane molecules. A further synthetic modification of Paclitaxel produced Docetaxel.

The World Of Microtubules And Cell Division

To understand how Docetaxel works, we must enter the world of tubulin, microtubules and cell division. Ultimately we wish to have the cell that takes in the chemo drug go into arrest, quite dividing, and die.

Tubulin is a globular protein that links together, like links forming a chain. The process is called polymerization and is similar to what occurs in plastic polymers and epoxy glues. There are several varieties of tubulin in the tubulin family and they are labeled α, β, γ, δ, and ϵ. It is the α- and β-tubulin (alpha- and beta-tubulin) that is largely at work in our cells and that is relevant concerning taxanes.

Cells polymerize the tubulin into chains, but it can also de-polymerize the chain. Depolymerizing the chain releases single tubulin proteins back into the cell microenvironment. The goal of the polymerization process is to form structural units within the cell called microtubules, a kind of cell skeleton. The players in the formation of microtubules are listed in **Table 9-2.**

Cells have a skeleton-like framework of protein, called the cytoskeleton. It consists of thin actin filaments, thicker keratin filaments, with the largest component being microtubules. Microtubules can assemble into bundles and these can even be used to propel cells. Microtubules give the cell structural support. Microtubules also have other functions and these are targets for PCa therapy, which we will describe shortly.

An important concept is that microtubules are not fixed length structures, but are dynamic and lengthen or shorten rapidly. This feature is a mode of action in our chemotherapy story, so we will go into this in some detail. Microtubules are short-lived lasting only a few minutes within the cell.

Table 9-2. **The players involved with microtubules and their role in cell division**.	
Tubulin	A globular protein in cells—a building block for microtubules
Microtubule	A chain of tubulin molecules that gives structure to cells. Used in mitosis
Mitosis	Cell division—a mother cell divides into two identical daughter cell
GTP → GDP	The triphosphate of Guanine, converting to its diphosphate version. Similar to ATP → ADP
Centrosome	A structure in a cell acting as an anchor that many microtubules attach to.
Mitotic spindle	A pair of opposing centrosomes with microtubules that are attached to DNA chromosomes and being pulled apart for cell division.

The basic unit of the polymer is a pair (dimer) of tubulin protein molecules; one an α-tubulin and the other a β-tubulin. These two stick together forming a peanut shaped complex called a tubulin (hetero) dimer. Each of the tubulin molecules of the dimer binds a GTP (Guanosine triphosphate) molecule. GTP is very similar to the energy molecule ATP but with guanine (G) instead of adenine (A) (recall the four molecules making up the DNA code consist of a A, T, G, and C). The tubulin pair binds strongly to the microtubule advancing the growth forward of the microtubule.

Here is where it gets tricky. Imagine a bus with passengers that want out at any stop and there is an impatient driver. At each stop the driver opens the door and new passengers get on but they block those trying to exit. This is repeated at each stop with the bus passenger count growing. This continues until a stop is reached where there are no or few new passengers trying to enter. The passenger count now shrinks since the lack of entering passengers allows those already on the bus to exit. Microtubules (**Figure 9-1**) grow in a similar manner; they grow or shrink depending on available molecules in the environment.

Figure 9-1. Microtubules. More details at: K Kinoshita et al., Trends in Cell Biology 12(6), 267-273 (2002).

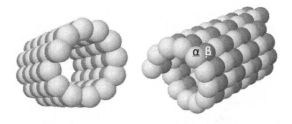

This is how it works. Tubulin is an enzyme and the GTP (note the T for tri) on the β-tubulin half of the tubulin-dimer is hydrolyzed to GDP (note the D, i.e. diphosphate), which means that one of the phosphate groups is cut off the molecule. This is similar to the energy currency molecule ATP being converted to ADP. When GTP is converted to GDP, the binding of the dimer to the microtubule is not as strong as it was previously with GTP. The end dimer wants off the "bus." The end tubulin-dimer may fall off the microtubule unless an additional tubulin-dimer attaches itself to the end to hold it in. The additional tubulin-dimer advances the polymer yet further. The added tubulin-dimer then has its GTP converted to GDP and so it now becomes loosely bound to the microtubule. It too needs to be secured by yet another additional GTP containing tubulin-dimer, which further advances growth. This continues as long as there are plenty of free-floating GTP-containing-tubulin-dimers circulating around the microtubule. If not, the tubulin-pairs begin falling off the end of the microtubule.

The situation of growing and shrinking microtubules based on the concentration of GTP containing tubulin dimers is called a "dynamic instability" and was discovered in 1984.

What has all this got to do with chemo drugs and cancer? Microtubules, by changing length, can apply push or pull forces on items within the cell. This plays a large part in mitosis where the cell divides into two. Replication is how tumors grow, so microtubule growth and retraction has everything to do with forces within cells which has everything to do with cell replication. Organizing centers called centrosomes act to anchor one end of the microtubule, while the other end is free to grow or retreat. The several-microtubule-bundle binding to the centrosome form a many-armed furry octopus-like structure (**Figure 9-2**). The microtubule is attached to the centrosome by a ring of tubulin, in this case γ-tubulin.

In preparation for mitosis (cell division), the centrosome splits into two forming anchoring points. The two move to opposite sides of the cell nucleus. These two form centers from which to pull material away into two groups that eventually become the two daughter cells of cell division. The membrane covering the nucleus disassembles and the microtubules grab hold of the chromosomes, which is the packaged DNA containing all the genes. By this time the chromosomes have themselves replicated forming a duplicate pair. A microtubule from each side attaches to one member of the chromosome pair. This structure is the mitotic spindle, which consists of two opposing centrosomes with their microtubules tugging on one chromosome in the pair. It is unbelievable that all this occurs; a truly miraculous sequence of events.

Figure 9-2. Cell division. Mitotic spindle consisting of microtubules anchored to centrosomes and tugging on chromosomes to separate them during the process of the cell dividing into two. This spectacular image illustrates that life is surely magical. Courtesy National Heart, Lung, and Blood Institute, National Institutes of Health, Nasser Rusan.

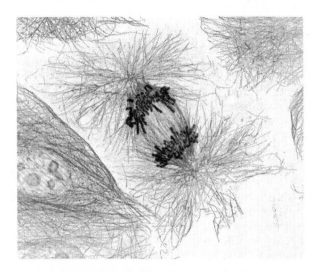

It is clear that microtubules are a key feature of the whole cell division picture. It is a division that we would not like to occur in prostate cancer cells.

Mode Of Action Of Docetaxel (Taxotere)

Docetaxel does its job by working on microtubules in the cell. Specifically it interferes with the function of the mitotic spindle, thus interrupting division of the cell. Tumors grow by cell division, so it is hoped that this stops the growth of tumors. But a temporary reprieve of growth is not enough. The cells that start to divide but cannot are induced into apoptosis, a programmed cell death. This not only stops tumor growth, but shrinks the existing tumor. That is, if it all goes according to the general mode of action.

The dynamic instability of microtubules is the target for agents like Docetaxel. The polymerization-depolymerization tug of war can be interfered with by drugs in one of two ways—promote polymerization by strengthening the interaction between tubulin dimers, or promote depolymerization by weakening the interaction. There are drugs that will do either. Docetaxel is a polymerization stabilizer. This was first discovered in test tube experiments in 1979.

Docetaxel does not bind well to a free tubulin dimer. It binds best to the dimer when it is part of a microtubule. It binds to the β-tubulin half of the dimer in a deep binding pocket that is at the interface with adjacent dimers. It is quite a different location from where GTP (or GDP) binds. When Docetaxel binds, it changes the structure of the β-tubulin by altering a loop within the protein. This conformational change strengthens the interaction of one dimer with its neighboring dimers in the microtubule. At the low concentration of Docetaxel that we use, it is not quite true to say that polymerization is enhanced, but rather that depolymerization becomes more difficult. Thus the microtubule is stronger so that the dynamical properties that are in full force during mitosis are altered. This alteration of the dynamics interferes with the population enhancing cell division event. The cell cycle is interrupted and apoptosis of the cell (hopefully) follows.

Does It Work On PCa? The Evidence

The TAX327 trial, reported in 2004, was an international effort lead by a researcher at University of Toronto, Canada. A total of 1,006 men were enrolled and contained three arms of approximately equal numbers. Each arm was chosen randomly and all patients had metastatic castrate resistant prostate cancer (mCRPC) and all were on androgen deprivation therapy. Mitoxantrone was commonly used for these patients at that time, which improved the quality of life but did not increase overall survival. (A short section on Mitoxantrone is given below.) The three arms were: (i) Mitoxantrone every 3 weeks (ii) 75mg/m^2 Docetaxel every three weeks, and (iii) 30mg/m^2 Docetaxel weekly for 5 of every 6 weeks. Note that the total dosages of arms (ii) and (iii) were the same but were administered over different periods of time. In addition, all three groups received Prednisone. Steroids, such as the corticosteroid Dexamethasone is often administered with taxanes and help alleviate allergic reactions and side effects.

Table 9-3. Tax327 Trial From IF Tannock et al., New England Journal of Medicine 351, 1502-1512 (2004).	Mitoxantrone	Docetaxel weekly	Docetaxel every 3 weeks
Survival Hazard ratio	1.00	0.91	0.76
Median survival time	16.5 months	17.4 months	18.9 months
>50% decrease in PSA serum	32%	48%	45%
Reduction in Pain	22%	31%	35%
Improved Quality of life	23%	23%	22%

Table 9-3 shows the results of the TAX327 trial comparing the three arms. The important line is that of median overall survival time, the primary endpoint of the study. Compared to the then standard of palliative care treatment of Mitoxantrone, there was an overall increase of

survival of 2.4 months, from 16.5 months to 18.9 months. It is not a huge increase. In these late-stage cancer patients, it is nothing close to a cure, but adds 2-3 months of life. The medical community refers to this as "significant improvement." I view it more as incremental improvement.

The overall survival curves (not shown) of the three arms in the TAX327 trial are fairly tight together—the differences are not huge. Adverse effects were more common in the Docetaxel groups, as Docetaxel has higher toxicity than Mitoxantrone. So the researchers commented that Mitoxantrone might still be appropriate for some patients where toxicity is a concern. That was the thinking in 2004.

At the same time as the results of the TAX327 trial came out, the results of the Southwest Oncology Group (SWOG) also came out (NCT00004001). The two reports were back-to-back in the New England Journal of Medicine in 2004. The Southwest Oncology Group trial was very similar to the TAX327 trial. This SWOG trial had just two arms and compared Docetaxel plus Estramustine to Mitoxantrone plus Prednisone. A total of 674 men participated, and the two arms were assigned randomly. The men had metastatic castrate resistant prostate cancer.

Estramustine is a derivative of estrogen and, like Docetaxel, acts on microtubules. But instead of favoring polymerization like Docetaxel, it favors depolymerization. This seems to be pushing and pulling at the same time, but the combination of the two is believed to produce a synergy making the combination more effective.

Table 9-4 shows the major results of the SWOG trial. In this case the median overall survival time from Docetaxel is increased by 1.9 months from 15.6 to 17.5 months. Again we find a modest increase in survival. Side effects were more common in the Docetaxel group.

Table 9-4. **SWOG trial**	Mitoxantrone	Docetaxel
Survival Hazard Ratio	1.00	0.80
Overall Median Survival	15.6 months	17.5 months
Median time to progression	3.2 months	6.3 months
>50% PSA decline	27%	50%

Blocking Androgen Receptors From Crossing The Nuclear Line Of Scrimmage

Docetaxel is a drug that targets tubulin. But as a bonus it appears to impair androgen receptors (ARs) from crossing from the outer region of the cell, the cytoplasm, into the data center, the nucleus. This halts the androgen receptor from producing transcriptional activity in the cell. In plain words, this means that AR-inducible genes like PSA within prostate cancer cells are expressed at a reduced level if we reduce AR crossing into the nucleus. To express genes, the activated androgen receptor must translocate from the outer portion of the cell across the nuclear membrane into the nucleus where the DNA is stored.

The result that Docetaxel inhibits AR translocation was found in a study published in 2010 centered at the University of Kentucky. The reduction of AR translocation was not huge but significant. The experiments were done in test tubes and two groups of cells were tested—those from Docetaxel treated patients and those from patients that had not been treated with Docetaxel. The patients had high risk but localized prostate cancer. The Docetaxel treatment was a secondary treatment (neoadjuvant) given before the patients underwent a prostatectomy.

It was found that in untreated cancer cells 50% of the ARs were in the cell nucleus, while in Docetaxel treated cells 38% of the ARs were in the nucleus. That's a 24% drop in nuclear AR; the nucleus is where the AR does its job. The total amount of androgen receptors in treated and untreated cells was about the same. So docetaxel was not reducing the number of ARs, it just hindered their ability to translocate into the nucleus. This reduction of nuclear AR should produce a reduction in AR inducible genes. One such gene is PSA. Indeed, the amount of PSA produced in Docetaxel treated and untreated PCa cells correlated with the number of nuclear androgen receptors.

Thus Docetaxel reduces PSA in PCa cells, it inhibits AR nuclear translocation and the number of ARs in the nucleus, and it inhibits the transcriptional activity of the AR. All of these are very positive results. But what does microtubules have to do with the androgen receptor? At first blush, the answer is nothing. But in living cells nothing is simple. We find that taxanes interfere with ARs translocating from the cytoplasm to the nucleus passing through the membrane separating the two. Microtubules are not directly needed for AR translocation. Also, taxanes do not modify the structure or composition of the AR that we know of. Only guesses can be made. A guess is that the ARs bind to microtubules and this somehow enables ARs to more easily cross into the nucleus. Taxanes increase the stability of microtubules and this interferes with microtubules aiding the AR to translocate.

An important detail from this work is that inhibition of AR translocation appears for both normal ARs and AR variants missing a ligand-binding domain. Recall that ARs without a ligand-binding domain have no place to bind androgen (the ligand) and are active without androgen. These variants appear in aggressive or very advanced PCa. It is good news that taxanes reduce translocation. If only taxanes were not so toxic in their side effects.

Drug Resistance

We acquire a drug resistance to chemotherapy drugs after repeated use. It seems surprising that cells can become resistant to a drug that targets microtubules. There are several mechanisms proposed for resistance to taxanes, although the exact cause is uncertain. Popular explanations include:

    (i)   Change in tubulin isotypes (not all tubulin is the same).

    (ii)   Efflux mechanisms (removal of taxanes).

    (iii) Alteration of cell death pathways.

    (iv) Mutations of tubulin that affect the polymerization and dynamics of microtubules.

Tubulin Isotypes — βIII-Tubulin: Not all β-tubulin is the same.

There are several variations (isotypes) of β-tubulin and they are denoted βI, βII, βIII, βIV, βV and so on. The one of particular interest is βIII. Usually there is very little βIII in our cells, but when they do show up, they are resistant to Docetaxel. We know that Docetaxel attaches to β-tubulin and changes its dynamics. But the assembly and dynamics of βIII-tubulin in microtubules is different from other isotypes.

    A study of 73 men in 2012 from the Henry Ford Hospital in Detroit indeed found evidence that βIII-tubulin in prostate cancer cells responded less to Docetaxel. How this was found is interesting. Men who had progressed to mCRPC were given Docetaxel and their progress followed. Men that have a prostatectomy have their prostate tissue archived by fixing in formalin and embedded with paraffin. The tissue of these men was examined for evidence of βIII-tubulin in their prostates, which were removed far earlier than their Docetaxel treatment. They did this by staining the tissue with an antibody. They were classified as either βIII+ or βIII-, depending on whether there was or was not any βIII-tubulin.

    Of the 73 patients followed, 26 (35%) were found to have βIII-tubulin in their tissue. **Table 9-5** shows that those with βIII-tubulin had a shorter overall survival time than those that did not, as well as a less positive PSA response.

    The TAX357 and SWOG trials had an increase in overall survival of 2.4 months and 1.9 months respectively. A little juggling of the results of **Table 9.5** also hints at an approximate 2-month increased survival time from Docetaxel, even though the raw data does not have a control

144

group of patients not receiving Docetaxel. To see a 2-month increased survival time for Docetaxel, let's make the bold assumption that Docetaxel had no benefit for the βIII+ group and categorize them as not having been given Docetaxel at all! Then the difference between the average patient (a random group receiving Docetaxel) and the βIII+ group (a group we pretend did not receive Docetaxel) is 2.3 months (19.1-16.8). This is very similar to the increase in overall survival from the two clinical trials. Perhaps we are playing with numbers, but it does illustrate that the assumption that patients with βIII+ have no docetaxel benefit is consistent with the results of rigorous clinical trials where patients include both βIII+ and βIII- subjects.

Table 9-5. **Henry Ford Hosp Study**	βIII+	βIII-	Average
Number of patients	26 (35%)	47 (65%)	
Median Overall Survival Time	16.8 months	20.4 months	19.1 months
Any PSA decline	65%	89%	81%
>50% PSA decline	52%	70%	64%

Efflux Mechanisms: You put money in your bank account, but it seems there are "pumps" to remove it just as fast as you put it in. Cells experience the same with biochemicals. Cells have mechanisms to pump out (efflux) material from within the cell to the outside. Taxanes enter the cell on one side, and may exit out the other side without performing their desired function. The pumps are proteins in the outer cell membrane that has channels for such removal. Transporter proteins bring their target cargo (e.g. Docetaxel) to the channel protein for removal. A class of cargo transporters of proteins is the ATP-binding cassette (ABC) transporters. One specific ABC transporter, P-glycoprotein, also known as Pgp, may become over-expressed and thus produce drug resistance. This clearly illustrates the complex fight we face. We need another drug to inhibit expression or functioning of Pgp without disturbing other functioning in the hope that resistance is due to efflux of Docetaxel, and in the hope that Docetaxel is actually providing benefit.

Alteration Of Cell Death Pathways:
Bcl-2 is an oncogen that inhibits cell death through apoptosis (cell suicide). This gene may be over-expressed due to taxanes. In addition, the resulting Bcl-2 protein can become phosphorylated which adds a PO_4^{3-} group to the protein. Phosphorylation is a common strategy for altering the functioning of proteins, particularly enzymes. Taxanes can lead to Bcl-2 protein becoming phosphorylated, which downstream leads to inhibition of cellular apoptosis.

Side Effects And Adverse Effects
There is a long laundry list of adverse effects and they can be serious. Sources specifically on this topic should be consulted. A very small fraction of patients cannot stand the chemotherapy treatment and can die from it. But the common adverse effects are nausea, fluid retention, and eyes watering (in the middle of the night). Neuropathy (loss of feeling in feet etc.) can be long lasting and is far too common. During treatment there is a general feeling of sickness and extreme tiredness. One also becomes susceptible to infection due to a reduced white blood count that compromises the immune system. Many people are allergic to taxanes. Your best-laid plans may need to be altered because of this. Other drugs are given to reduce the potential for allergic symptoms.

Early Treatment With Docetaxel?
Docetaxel was traditionally given as a kind of last resort, because of its toxicity. The original FDA approval was for metastatic castrate resistant prostate cancer. Indeed, many of the new drug therapies are for the castrate resistant form of PCa. When it becomes castrate resistant, the cancer cells have mutated to become more aggressive and more

difficult to treat. A legitimate question to ask then is "Why wait until the cancer becomes castrate resistant?"

That is a question I ask often. Part of the answer unfortunately is that insurance often will not pay for drugs not FDA approved for a specific indication. The first test-bed of powerful anti-cancer drugs are on severe patients where we are going for broke.

In June of 2014 at the annual American Society of Clinical Oncology (ASCO) meeting in Chicago, the results of a trial on early Docetaxel administration were presented. The study was led by Christopher J. Sweeney, a medical oncologist at the Lank Center of Genitourinary Oncology at the Dana-Farber Cancer Institute in Boston. The study was the highlight of the prostate cancer portion of the meeting. I was fortunate enough to attend the session.

It was a phase III trial (CHAARTED trial, NCT00309985) and involved men who were still hormone sensitive (not castrate resistant) and had recently been found to have metastasized disease. The trial compared men that went on androgen deprivation therapy (ADT) and those on ADT plus Docetaxel. For those getting chemotherapy, the chemo was started within 4 months of starting ADT. It is not clear how important this is, and what effect significant delays in starting chemotherapy might have. The Docetaxel treatment was every 3 weeks for 6 cycles, with a dosage of $75mg/m^2$. The two arms were randomized and had roughly equal numbers of patients. The primary endpoint of the trial was overall survival. Men were enrolled between 2006 and 2012, and the median follow-up was 29 months. The average age was 63.

Analysis of the data classified men as having either low volume or high volume disease. High volume disease was considered for those with metastases to internal organs (visceral disease) or having four or more bone metastases. About 2/3 of the patients had high volume disease.

The Early Docetaxel Trial of **Table 9-6** shows the results. Median overall survival of those with high volume disease is dramatically increased by 17 months (32.2 mo *vs.*

49.2 months). By prostate cancer standards this is huge. Certainly it is expected that those with low volume disease live longer than those with high volume disease. The median was not reached for the low volume disease subpopulation because of the relatively short follow-up time of the trial.

Table 9-6. CHAARTED Early Docetaxel Trial	ADT only	ADT + Docetaxel
Number of patients	393	397
Percent with high volume disease	64%	67%
Median Overall Survival High volume disease.	32.2 months	49.2 months
Median Overall Survival Low volume disease	Not reached	Not reached

Early docetaxel remains controversial. At the 2015 ASCO meeting, one year after the 2014 meeting where early docetaxel was promoted, Dr. M Hussain argued for early treatment (for high volume disease), while Dr. H Scher argued that it be given late. Part of the controversy stems from a second trial, GETUG-AFU 15, which was smaller and not as favorable for early application of Docetaxel.

A Little History: Mitoxantrone

The first chemotherapy drug approved by the FDA for CRPC was Mitoxantrone (Novantrone). The drug was approved in 1996 and is used in combination with a corticosteroid (Prednisone). That was nearly 20 years ago and it illustrates how crude things were for PCa. Mitoxantrone offers no survival benefit, but is palliative and may relieve pain in some patients, improving the quality of life. The study that led to FDA approval was Canadian and it found just 29% of patients experienced a positive palliative response. Cardiac toxicity is reported in some patients.

The mode of action of Mitoxantrone is quite

different than the modern taxane chemotherapy drugs. It is useful to review how it works. Cell division again is a target, and acts by preventing DNA replication during cell division. Its target is a somewhat miraculous enzymatic machine called topoisomerase. We get clues to how topoisomerase works from the word itself. Topo refers to topology, the geometry of the molecule, an isomer is a molecule identical to another molecule, and the suffix "ase" denotes an enzyme. Before cell division occurs, the DNA of the cell must be replicated. But the DNA is not lying out flat, but is knotted up and coiled much like a long outdoor power cord thrown into a heap. When DNA is replicated, we now have two entangled DNA double helices. The job is not to unknot either one, but to free one DNA from the other. The molecules are so long that the ends cannot be treaded through the knots to untangle them as we might do with a power cord. One of the two DNA molecules has to be cut, passed through the second DNA, then the cut DNA must be mended back together. We have no machine that could do such a complex job say with power cords, but our bodies do it each time our cells divide. Still think life is not a miracle?

So what exactly does Mitoxantrone do? This drug inserts itself in the groove of DNA double helix, a process called intercalation. This interferes with the action of the topoisomerase, so that the replication of the DNA is stalled. But the process of cell division is well underway, but it cannot be completed. This causes the cell to die. There is nothing specific about cancer cells in this description. This can act on any cell. This is part of the reason chemo drugs are so toxic. Of course, cancer cells are highly prolific and divide rapidly, so they are more vulnerable to cell division interference.

Cabazitaxel (Jevtana)

Cabazitaxel is a taxane drug that is used as a "second line" chemotherapy. Docetaxel is the first line, but repeated use leads to resistance. The question then is, how to get around this resistance. A search was made for drugs that were similar to Docetaxel but did not have the affinity for the ABC transporter P-glycoprotein (Pgp). Recall that Pgp is an ATP dependent efflux pump that removes drugs from the cell. This is one important mode of chemo-resistance. Docetaxel enters the cell, and the cell pumps it back out. But to be pumped out, it needs to bind to Pgp. Cabazitaxel has properties similar to Docetaxel, but does not bind as well to Pgp. Once PCa was considered hormone refractory and chemotherapy resistant, now we know it is neither at least in many cases.

Cabazitaxel is a taxane so its mode of action is on microtubules, similar to the action of Docetaxel. Its structure is similar to Docetaxel and Paclitaxel. It is semi-synthetic in that it has substitutions and additions made to the 3-ring core to make it more potent and not attracted to Pgp efflux pumps. The chemical formula of Cabazitaxel is $C_{48}H_{63}NO_{15}$ vs. $C_{43}H_{53}NO_{14}$ for Docetaxel. The drug was first studied (then called XRP6258, TX0258, or RPR116258A) in cell lines in test tubes and found to be as potent as Docetaxel.

Does Cabazitaxel Work?

The FDA in June 2010 approved Cabazitaxel with Prednisone for mCRPC for those previously treated with Docetaxel. Cabazitaxel has activity in both Docetaxel-sensitive and Docetaxel-resistant scenarios.

A randomized Phase-3 trial for men with progressive disease after Docetaxel was reported in 2010. It was multi-national with leadership from Sutton, UK, and Tulane, New Orleans. Half of the patients received Mitoxantrone and half received Cabazitaxel. The trial had two arms. One arm received Prednisone plus intravenous Mitoxantrone ($12mg/m^2$) and the other arm received Prednisone plus intravenous Cabazitaxel ($25mg/m^2$). The trial was designed for patients to receive 10 rounds spaced 3 weeks apart.

Previous trials found that lowering the white blood cell count (neutropenia) is the primary dose limiting toxicity. The primary end point was overall survival and secondary end points were progression free survival and tumor response rate. Enrollment of the 755 patients was between 1/2007-10/2008, and they were followed for a median time of 12.8 months.

A summary of the important results is shown in **Table 9-7**. There was an increase in overall survival by 2.3 months in favor of the Cabazitaxel arm, which resulted in a hazard ratio for death of 0.79. It is not huge but something. Most patients did not have a reduction in tumor load, as the tumor response rate was low in both arms. Also the progression free survival time was not long in either arm, but the Cabazitaxel arm's time was twice that of the mitoxantrone arm.

Table 9-7. UK/Tulane Trial	Mitoxantrone	Cabazitaxel
Median Overall Survival	12.7 months	15.1 months
Tumor response rate	4.4%	14.4%
Median Progression Free survival	1.4 months	2.8 months

Neutropenia was common adverse effect with 82% of those on Cabazitaxel experiencing it. Also, 8% of patients on Cabazitaxel had both fever and neutropenia (febrile neutropenia).

Neuroendocrine PCa And Platinum Chemotherapy

There are particularly aggressive variants of PCa called small cell carcinoma or also described as neuroendocrine prostate cancer. Recall that neuroendocrine cells are a variety of cells within the prostate, and aggressive prostate cancer variants express markers like those of neuroendocrine differentiated cells. These aggressive variants are especially difficult to treat, and the outcomes are not as favorable as those of other prostate cancer cells. They are usually treated with a different form of chemotherapy—a platinum-based chemotherapy.

In 1965, physicist Barnett Rosenberg at Michigan State University was playing Dr. Frankenstein. He applied electric and magnetic fields at radio frequencies to bacterial cells *E. coli*. The goal was to determine if these fields played a role in cell division. Immersed in the cell culture medium were platinum electrodes to which the voltage was applied. Platinum is a commonly used electrode material (but very expensive) since it is usually non-reactive in an aqueous environment.

E. Coli is a single cell critter, so each time the cell divides it doubles its number. Thus cell division is easy to determine. The Frankenstein experiment showed that in the electromagnetic field, *E. Coli* bacterial cells elongated themselves up to 300 times their normal length. Certainly strange—but they stopped dividing. The inhibition of cell division was not a result of the electromagnetic field, but turned out rather to be due to the "inert" platinum (Pt). It had formed a compound $Pt(NH_3)_2Cl_2$ in the bacterial culture which stopped cell division. This compound is Cisplatin, and thus began the development of platinum based chemotherapy drugs, called platins.

The platin family of chemotherapy drugs includes Cisplatin, Carboplatin, Oxaliplatin, Satraplatin and Picoplatin. The other platins were developed in time by altering the Cisplatin molecule to reduce toxicity, ease of use (e.g. oral *vs.* intravenous), or to fight chemo-resistance. Cisplatin is toxic to the kidneys and carboplatin was developed to reduce this toxicity. Cisplatin is used on many forms of cancer—prostate cancer is just one application.

The mode of action of platin drugs is reminiscent of that of Mitoxantrone in that platins interfere with DNA processes. Cisplatin covalently binds to DNA (called an adduct). Usually Cisplatin will bind to nitrogen on the guanine (guanine is the G in the DNA A-T-G-C code) and less frequently to nitrogen on adenine (A). It usually binds to two of these bases, either within the same strand in the

152

double helix, or it cross-links the two strands together. In simple terms it glues-up the DNA. There is a major disruption of the DNA molecule, which causes local changes in its configuration (amount of helical twist, bend etc.). Maintenance proteins recognize this change as an aberration or damage. DNA damage proteins are recruited to fix the problem, which is difficult to fix. Repair pathways and cell arrest pathways are alerted; the result is to trigger is cell death by apoptosis.

In the mid-2000s it was looking like Satraplatin might be FDA approved for CRPC. But disappointing overall survival results were found, and the drug is currently not FDA approved. There is less known about how to best treat small cell prostate carcinoma than the "usual" prostate cancer. A recent study in 2013 from The University of Texas MD Anderson Center incorporated a two front approach. The first front combined Carboplatin and Docetaxel followed by a second-line combination of Etoposide and Cisplatin. Etoposide is a topoisomerase inhibitor, whose action we recall is the basis of the mode of action of Mitoxantrone. So we can understand the rationale of this two front approach. The Carboplatin+Docetaxel fights cell division and replication on two fronts—the carboplatin acts on the DNA and the Docetaxel works on the microtubules. Both arrest cell division and can lead to cell death. Carboplatin is used instead of Cisplatin due to its reduced toxicity. Upon progression, the second front of Etoposide+Cisplatin is used. The Etoposide acts to prevent DNA replication during cell division by inhibiting the topoisomerase machine, while Cisplatin glues-up the DNA. This protocol covers a lot of bases and hopefully will provide benefit. If only there were no side effects.

References

Targeting Microtubules by Natural Agents for Cancer Therapy, E Mukhtar, VM Adhami, and H Mukhtar, Molecular Cancer Therapeutics 13(2), 275-284 (2014).

Dynamic instability of microtubule growth, T Mitchison and M Kirschner, Nature 312, 237-242 (1984).

Docetaxel plus Prednisone or Mitoxantrone plus Prednisone for Advanced Prostate Cancer, IF Tannock, R de Wit, WR Berry, J Horti, A Pluzanska, KN Chi, S Oudard, C Théodore, ND James, I Turesson, MA Rosenthal, and MA Eisenberger, for the TAX327 Investigators, New England Journal of Medicine 351(15), 1502-1512 (2004).

Docetaxel and Estramustine Compared with Mitoxantrone and Prednisone for Advanced Refractory Prostate Cancer, DP Petrylak, CM Tangen, MHA Hussain, PN Lara, Jr., JA Jones, ME Taplin, PA Burch, D Berry, C Moinpour, Manish Kohli, MC Benson, EJ Small, D Raghavan, and ED Crawford, New England Journal of Medicine 351(15), 1513-1520 (2004).

Tubulin-Targeting Chemotherapy Impairs Androgen Receptor Activity in Prostate Cancer, M-L Zhu, CM Horbinski, M Garzotto, DZ Qian, TM Beer, and N Kyprianou, Cancer Research 70(20), 7992-8002 (2010).

βIII-tubulin expression as a predictor of docetaxel resistance in metastatic castrate-resistant prostate cancer, BE Sanchez. N Gupta, M Mahan, ER Barrack, P Reddy and C Hwang, Journal of Clinical Oncology 30, supplement e15174 (2012) [2012 Annual meeting ASCO].

Impact on overall survival (OS) with chemohormonal therapy versus hormonal therapy for hormone-sensitive newly metastatic prostate cancer (mPrCa): An ECOG-led phase III randomized trial, C Sweeney, Y-H Chen, MA Carducci, et al., ASCO Annual Meeting. Abstract LBA2, Presented June 1, 2014.

All tangled up: how cells direct, manage and exploit topoisomerase function, SM Vos, EM Tretter, BH Schmidt and JM Berger, Nature Reviews Molecular Cell Biology 12, 827-841 (2011).

Cabazitaxel, MD Galsky, A Dritselis, P Kirkpatrick and WK Oh, Nature Reviews Drug Discovery, 9 677-678 (2010).

Prednisone plus cabazitaxel or mitoxantrone for metastatic castration-resistant prostate cancer progressing after docetaxel treatment: a randomised open-label trial, JS de Bono, S Oudard, M Ozguroglu, S Hansen, J-P Machiels, I Kocak, G Gravis, I Bodrogi, MJ Mackenzie, L Shen, M Roessner, S Gupta and AO Sartor, for the TROPIC Investigators, Lancet 376, 1147-1154 (2010).

Inhibition of cell division in Escherichia coli by electrolysis products from an platinum electrode, B Rosenberg, L van Camp and T Krigas, Nature 205, 698-699 (1965).

The resurgence of platinum-based cancer chemotherapy, L Kelland, Nature Reviews Cancer 7, 573-584 (2007).

Platinum-Based Chemotherapy for Variant Castrate-Resistant Prostate Cancer, AM Aparicio, AL Harzstark, PG Corn, S Wen, JC Araujo, S-M Tu, LC Pagliaro, J Kim, RE Millikan, CJ Ryan, NM Tannir, AJ Zurita, P Mathew, W Arap, P Troncoso, PF Thall, and CJ Logothetis, Clinical Cancer Research 19(13), 3621–3630 (2013).

Chapter 10

The Conflicting Case to Reduce Trouble – Metformin

Mavericks once played an essential role in research. Indeed, their worked defined the 20th century. We must relearn how to support them... . From a 2014 letter to *The Guardian* signed by 30 scientists including 3 Nobel laureates.

Science sometimes sends mixed signals. The case of the use of generic drug Metformin for prostate cancer is our poster child for this. Metformin is a drug given to diabetic patients to control their blood sugar. It also goes by the name Glucophage, which translates to glucose (sugar) eater. So what has this to do with prostate cancer? That is what we will explore on our Lewis and Clark expedition in this chapter. There is evidence both ways on the use of Metformin on PCa—evidence that it potentially can produce great things in advanced PCa, and evidence that it does nothing. But even PCa drugs that are proven to "work," are not effective for every patient. Metformin has been proposed to be a treatment for other forms of cancer, as well as prostate cancer. On the plus side, Metformin is inexpensive, has relatively few side effects, is well studied (for other diseases), and is familiar to physicians. One side effect to watch out for is lactic acidosis. It is rare but an important side effect. Metformin is not FDA approved for prostate cancer.

Metformin is a small molecule of just 20 atoms, with the chemical formula $C_4N_5H_{11}$. It is a derivative of the molecule biguanide, $C_2N_5H_7$. It is primarily used to control blood sugar in type-2 diabetes. This turned out to be useful in discovering its benefits concerning prostate cancer since there is a significant subset of prostate cancer sufferers that also have diabetes. We can see if they do better than your run-of-the-mill prostate cancer patient.

Oxygen, Hypoxia, and Hypoxia Inducible Factors

A **suggested** mode of action of Metformin for prostate cancer relates to oxygen. Oxygen and its role in cancer is also a somewhat controversial subject. In 1956, Otto Warburg published an important paper in the journal Science, "*On the origin of Cancer cells.*" His hypothesis is that cancer is caused by an injury of the respiration system of cancer cells. Respiration produces energy to power cells. When this energy source is compromised, cells either die or find another energy source. Otto Warburg suggested that a fermentation pathway replaces respiration. He is no quack. People listened since he received the 1931 Nobel Prize in Physiology/Medicine "for his discovery of the nature and mode of action of the respiratory enzyme." He had been working on the respiration question in tumors for a long time including his book "*On metabolism of tumors,*" originally in German but reprinted in English in 1930.

Respiration is the process of burning hydrocarbons to produce carbon dioxide (the gas that comprises bubbles in soda pop) and water. The burning of glucose ($C_6H_{12}O_6$) is

$$C_6H_{12}O_6 + 6O_2 + 6H_2O \rightarrow 12H_2O + 6\,CO_2$$

The point of this discussion is that the process requires oxygen that we get from the air we breathe and is supplied to blood through the lungs. The competing fermentation process does not require oxygen.

Generally, cancer cells need oxygen to grow. That is the origin of angiogenesis, the growth of new blood vessels to the regions of tumors. Blood vessels are needed to produce an abundant oxygen supply to feed the growing tumor's needs. Cancer cells may produce a signaling molecule named vascular endothelial growth factor (VEGF). These growth factors cause more blood vessels to be produced.

Fast growing tumors may run out of oxygen, producing a local state of oxygen starvation, called hypoxia. But cancer has control systems it uses to remedy the situation. One of these mechanisms is that cells undergoing hypoxia produce hypoxia inducible factors (HIFs). Inhibiting HIFs is a potential target for an anti-cancer therapy. And that is how oxygen ties in with the Metformin story. Cells become more aggressive with HIFs as these are emergency signals to the cells. Stress induces other factors to come into play and they will use these other factors to survive.

One might conjecture that it may be better to have given the cancer cells enough oxygen in the first place. But who knows. There is a following of believers that cancer hates oxygen, although I am not one of them. One can increase the blood supply by increasing the diameter of the blood vessels; that is, dilating them. There are vasodilators molecules that do this. One of them is nitric oxide, simply a nitrogen and an oxygen atom, NO. Nitroglycerine, also called glycerol trinitrate (GTN) to make you forget that nitroglycerine is also used in explosives, is also used, as it produces NO in the body. Heart patients take GTN.

The protein hypoxia-inducible factor, HIF1a (HIF1 alpha), is expressed in prostate cells undergoing oxygen starvation (hypoxia). It is a defense mechanism against the oxidative stress, and may also be up-regulated from other purposely-applied stresses such as ADT, radiation, or chemotherapy. Under stress, it is believed that prostate cancer cells react by becoming more aggressive. Additionally, androgen receptors, the receptors that bind androgen and signal the cell to grow, are up-regulated by HIF1a. A reasonable hypothesis then is that a chemical inhibitor of HIF1a will reduce the aggressiveness of prostate cancer as it struggles for a better blood supply, or as we apply stresses to it from prostate cancer therapies. However, there are no specifically targeted inhibitors of HIF1a, rather nonspecific inhibitors that have other primary targets (cardiac or type-2 diabetes therapies) but additionally inhibit HIF1a. Metformin is a non-specific inhibitor. Finally, I hope it is clear that discussing a mode of action of Metformin for prostate cancer must be read with caution. We are not even sure Metformin has benefit for PCa patients, so assuming the hypoxia mode of action is correct is uncertainty piled on top

158

of uncertainty.

Evidence

There is evidence pro and con for metformin and its benefit for PCa sufferers. But one must be careful what the question is. The question might be "Does Metformin help prevent prostate cancer?" or the question might be "Does Metformin provide a benefit for those who already have (advanced) prostate cancer?" The answers to these questions may differ significantly. We will primarily focus on the later question, specifically for advanced prostate cancer.

A recent piece of significant positive evidence comes from Australia in a study reported in 2014 by Ranasinghe and coworkers. This was a retrospective study of 98 prostate cancer patients from 1983-2011. The retrospective nature of the study here means that they went through hospital records of PCa patients that fit the criteria of the study. This contrasts with the gold standard, a prospective study, in which patients are recruited with controllable conditions being met. The patients in the retrospective study were those at a hospital in Melbourne, Australia. The trial compared PCa patients taking an HIF1a inhibitor with those not taking one. The inhibitors were of 3 types and were taken either for cardiac problems or type-2 diabetes. The three inhibitors were Digoxin (cardiac), Metformin (diabetes), and Angiotensin-2 receptor blocker (cardiac). They were taking inhibitors not for cancer but for cardiac problems or diabetes. Those not taking an HIF1a inhibitor are considered a control group, and are compared to the HIF1a inhibitor group. The group taking the inhibitor was small, with only 18 patients taking non-specific inhibitors of HIF1a. The small number of patients is a major negative for this study.

Although a small study, and although a retrospective study (two strikes against it), the results are quite impressive. There were two major findings. One concerns the time to progress from hormone sensitive to hormone-refractory (castrate sensitive to castrate resistant), and the other concerning the time to metastasize. The median time (50%

occurrence) to castrate resistance and to metastases are
shown in the **Table 10-1**.

Table 10-1. **2014 Retrospective Study, Austin Hospital, Melbourne, Australia**		
	No HIF1a inhibitors (N=66) , <Age>=64	HIF1a Inhibitors (N=18), <Age>=70
Median time to castrate resistance	2.7 years	6.7 years
Median metastases free survival time	2.6 years	5.1 years

We discuss these two findings in turn. The first
finding concerned the progression from hormone-sensitive
cancer to hormone-refractory cancer. Most new drug
therapies are applied to castrate resistant cancer, which is
when the cancer is far more difficult to treat. A drug to
prolong the hormone-sensitive state is much needed, as there
are no drug therapies that specifically target extending the
hormone-sensitive state. The median time to progression in
the control group (no inhibitor) was 2.7 years, while median
time to progression for those taking an inhibitor was 6.7
years. That is 4 years difference. Not 4 months, but 4 years.
The only other therapy that has a benefit anything like that is
the ADT therapy itself. The modern "wonder-drugs" for
CRPC have overall survival benefits of

* Abiraterone   (3.9 months -- Cougar Trial)
* Enzalutamide (4.8 months -- AFFIRM Trial)
* Sipuleucel-T (4.1 months – IMPACT Trial).

Overall survival and castrate resistant survival are different
things, but the point surly is not missed—extending the time
to castrate resistance by four years (if this result is actually
true) is a remarkable result and requires that PCa patients

and researchers take notice.

The second major finding concerned the time for the prostate cancer to metastasize. The median time of metastasis free survival is 2.6 years in the control group and 5.1 years in the group taking nonspecific HIF1a inhibitors.

The study also examined tissue samples of the prostates that they obtained from both groups. There were only four such samples in the inhibitor-taking group, and these four by chance were all taking Metformin. Staining the tissue with dyes to reveal HIF1a protein shows that the control group had higher HIF1a levels than the inhibitor-taking group. This indeed shows that the inhibitor-taking group was expressing reduced levels of HIF1a protein.

The results are very encouraging, but are they believable? The study was NOT prospective, starting with patients and randomizing them into two groups. This study was retrospective and there could be an unknown bias in the two groups. Those taking HIF1a inhibitors were not taking it because of cancer but for other ailments and for some unaccounted reason this could be the reason that led to better cancer outcomes for these patients. The small number (18) of patients taking inhibitors is a large reason for concern. All patients (in both groups) eventually received chemotherapy later in their treatment, and this too may be a bias in that these patients are likely to be more fit than average. The three drugs used all had a side-reaction in that they inhibited HIF1a, but this does not prove that this was the true cause of the positive response.

The evidence presented suggests that patients taking a nonspecific HIF1a inhibitor were able to delay the progression from hormone sensitive to hormone-refractory for those patients on continuous ADT. It also suggests that metastasis is delayed. If this new therapy is ever proven to be effective, it has advantages. The inhibitors are well known in the medical profession and their adverse effects are well characterized. They have generic forms, so they are not outrageously expensive like the newer cancer drugs. This however presents problems. A drug like Metformin is generic, so there is no motivation, for example, for a hungry startup to investigate its use in prostate cancer. Big pharmaceuticals also would not be interested. It comes down to fundamental research organizations like Universities and the NIH to lead the way on this one.

The first clinical data to show the benefit of a non-specific inhibitor was work from the Memorial-Sloan Kettering Cancer Center (MSKCC) in New York. This retrospective study was published in 2013. This study compiled data from 2,901 patients between 1992 and 2008 at MSKCC. The design studied the effect of one drug, Metformin, prescribed for type-2 diabetes. The patients had undergone external beam radiation therapy (EBRT) for localized PCa. Lymph node or distant metastasis patients were not included in the study. The data from patients was binned into three groups—non-diabetic patients, diabetics taking Metformin, and diabetics but not taking Metformin. This study had plenty of patients, but again, it too was retrospective.

The number of patients in the three groups was very different. The diabetic group taking Metformin group had 157 patients, the non-Metformin diabetic group had 162, and the non-diabetic group had 2,582 patients. Median follow up was 8.7 years. Those binned into the Metformin group could have started Metformin at any time while they were followed. This is a problem as we will see. This means they could have been taking it at PCa diagnosis, or started taking Metformin for diabetes while well into their journey with PCa.

A summary of the results is this—the diabetic group not taking Metformin had the worst prostate cancer results, but the diabetic group taking Metformin had better prostate cancer outcomes than the non-diabetic group. Thus Metformin appears to make up for the negative of having two diseases and this group surpassed those with no diabetic disease.

Let's look specifically at the outcomes. **Table 10-2** show the results for percentage of patients who experienced

(i) PSA progression (AKA biochemical failure), (ii) distant metastases, (iii) death from prostate cancer and (iv) castrate resistance. One notices that the diabetic group not taking Metformin had the worse outcomes, while the diabetic group taking Metformin had the best prostate cancer outcomes.

This study also is retrospective so we must remain skeptical. In particular, in isolation this study could be the result of some unaccountable benefit that diabetes and Metformin has on prostate cancer outcomes. But in light of the 2014 study where heart patients were included, it appears

Table 10-2. **2014 Retrospective study of Metformin use (Memorial Sloan-Kettering Cancer Center)**			
	Diabetic No Metformin (N=162)	Non-Diabetic (N=2582)	Diabetic With Metformin (N=157)
PSA Progression (Biochemical Failure)	32.7%	25.8%	16.5%
Developed Distant Metastases	24.1%	11.5%	5.7%
Death from PCa	13.0%	6.8%	1.9%
Developed castrate resistance (After Biochemical Failure)	43%	26%	4.0%

that the affect is not a result of diabetes + Metformin, but rather of the nonspecific $HIF1\alpha$ inhibitor (in this case Metformin).

Now we head into some controversy. A criticism of this study by a Canadian group led by Prof. Azoulay was that the immortal time bias likely produced these results. Immortal time bias is the same bias used when one states that Oscar award winners live longer than the general population. That statement is true. Oscar winners due live longer than the general population. The reason is not because an Oscar somehow actually makes you live longer (for example by removing stress), but because Oscar winners are generally already 30 or 40 or 50 years old when they win the award. Someone that has already made it to say 40 years old will likely live longer than an "average" person which also includes newborn or youngsters—the newborn and youngsters must survive childhood diseases, reckless teenage driving and parties, military service, and so on. The bias for the Metformin study is that patients were included in the Metformin-use bin even if they had first taken Metformin far after being diagnosed with prostate cancer. They made it quite some way without Metformin but now Metformin gets the credit. The MSKCC group responded to this criticism stating that they do not believe immortal time bias is a significant issue and note that only 18% of the Metformin group was not on Metformin from the beginning. Also, only 8% initiated Metformin after 3 years. The results were reanalyzed comparing the two diabetic groups—Metformin *vs.* non-Metformin. The hazard ratio of the two groups was similar to what it was before, but slightly less impressive, after reanalysis. Unfortunately the reanalysis was not between the Metformin group and the group without diabetes (and no Metformin). This is the far more interesting comparison. Also a reanalysis was not made for the time to progression to castrate resistance for those with biochemical failure, a key feature. For if we can delay (or stop) progression to CRPC, survival and quality of life is improved for PCa patients. I am deeply disappointed in that the interesting results of this study may (or may not) be compromised.

It is worth mentioning that the hypothesis of the MSKCC is not that metformin is an HIF1α inhibitor, but rather that it activates an adenosine monophosphate-activated protein kinase pathway (AMPK). This inhibits the MTOR (mammalian target of rapamycin) signaling. Lack of AMPK activation advances cell growth. But since there is uncertainty that Metformin has benefits in patients with PCa, there is even greater uncertainty to its mechanism of action. In fact, there are a multitude of suggested modes of action.

An interesting result was presented at the annual American Society of Clinical Oncology (ASCO) meeting in June 2015. It is a poster presented by scientists from Rutgers University to other scientists for comment and discussion, so should be considered preliminary. The lead scientist is Grace Lu-Yao. It was a population-based study (another retrospective study) that examined metformin use in prostate cancer patients who did or did not also take Statin drugs. Statin drugs are taken to control high cholesterol. The population included 22,110 high-risk prostate cancer patients, and data was extracted from prostate cancer patient Medicare statistics. Of this population 4,481 took statins alone, 1,356 took both Statins and Metformin, and 471 took Metformin alone. Notice that those that took Metformin, three-fourths of them also took Statins. That is a confounding factor for the study of Metformin if there ever was one.

This population study raises the possibility that the health benefits attributed to Metformin may be coming from Statins instead. A hazard ratio (HR) gives the ratio of the median survival time compared to no (or some other) treatment, [HR=(survival time while on drug)/(survival time no drug)]. In this study we have hazard ratios comparing patients that are drug takers with non-Metformin-non-Statin patients. A hazard ration of 2 means the rate of death is twice as large on the drug (a very bad thing), while a hazard ratio of 0.5 means the rate is one half for those taking the drug (obviously a very good thing). The drug takers and their HRs were (i) Metformin alone [HR=0.92], (ii) Statins alone [HR=0.60] and (iii) Metformin+Statin [HR=0.57]. This appears to indicate that the Statin drug is the effective drug for this population, and not Metformin. The study concludes that further studies investigate this. Our Lewis and Clark expedition is going through some very muddy water.

Finally we mention the results of an exploratory Phase 2 trial from Switzerland led by Dr. Rothermundt

(NCT01243385). The previous studies mentioned were retrospective. Finally, the Swiss trial gives us a true Phase 2 trial! It was a small trial of 44 men with progressive metastatic castrate resistant prostate cancer (mCRPC). All men came from Swiss centers and none were diabetic and had never previously taken Metformin. Patients received 1000mg of Metformin twice daily (2000mg/day). There was no control group. The primary goal of the trial was very modest—for 35% of the patients to achieve no disease progression for 12 weeks.

The major results of the trial were that (i) 36% of patients were progression free at 12 weeks (meeting the primary goal of the trial), (ii) 52% of patients had an increase in the PSA doubling time after taking Metformin, and (iii) 9% were progression free at 24 weeks. The researchers concluded that the Metformin in non-diabetic PCa patients is safe, yields a positive PSA response, may stabilize disease, and PSA doubling times were prolonged in some patients. These results are positive but very modest. But the i's are dotted and the t's crossed as this was a gold-standard prospective trial. One may infer from these results for mCRPC that Metformin is not a stand-alone drug, but may best be used in combination with other therapies. Since patients in this trial were already castrate resistant, the results of this trial do not address the very important question of delaying the onset of castrate resistance in the first place.

At the beginning of 2015, a clinicaltrials.gov search of "Metformin" AND "prostate cancer" yielded 14 clinical trials in various stages. For the related case of "metformin" AND "breast cancer" 30 clinical trials are listed. There is interest and action on the use of Metformin in both prostate and breast cancers. It will be some time before we know the results. One need not participate in a clinical trial to use Metformin however. It is available now and can be used off-label (meaning for a condition it is not approved). This is something your physician must decide. Clinical trials however, are the only way to find out what really works and won't kill you.

We have shown some evidence that Metformin has positive effects on PCa. But I emphatically remind the reader that there are plenty of reports that indicate Metformin has no or little benefit. I will just mention a couple. As they say at the end of far too many medical research reports, "more research is needed."

First a group from Wheeling Jesuit University in early 2015 reported on whether Metformin use had any affect on the diagnosis of PCa in patients. The patients in this retrospective study had undergone a biopsy and correlations were sought between the severity of the cancer found in the biopsy and previous Metformin use. About half of the patients were diagnosed by their biopsy to have PCa. They compared three groups — non-diabetic men, diabetic men not taking metformin, and diabetic men taking metformin. The overall conclusion was that PCa incidence, Gleason score or disease volume we not affected by Metformin usage.

In a second example, a Mayo Clinic study in 2014, examined the effect of Metformin on prostate cancer outcomes after radical prostatectomy. It was a retrospective study where the researchers examined the records of 12,052 patients who had undergone a radical prostatectomy and followed them for 5.1 years. Of these patients, 323 were diabetic taking Metformin, and 562 were diabetic and not taking Metformin. This study should be able to detect an effect of Metformin on established cases of PCa if there is one, and if unknown confounding effects do not kill the correlation. The conclusion of this study was that after a radical prostatectomy, that Metformin had no effect on disease production.

A Metformin Cocktail

The question of drug combinations is a difficult one as the number of possibilities grows rapidly. Should it be A with B, A with C, B with C and so on? But we are fortunate that even in these early days of the use of Metformin for prostate cancer that advances have been made in combining

Metformin with other drugs.

A second drug that has been found to be especially beneficial is the Polo-like kinase 1 (Plk1) inhibitor. The specific Plk1-inhibitor has the forgettable name BI2536. A very powerful synergy has been found in the combination of Metformin and BI2536 acting on PCa. However, it is early on in the detective story and its synergistic benefits have only been investigated (as of Jan. 2015) in test tubes and in mice. The work was reported Jan. 2015 and was performed at Purdue University and was led by Xiaoqi Liu. There have not yet been any clinical trials in humans on the Metformin plus BI2536 cocktail.

Kinases are enzymes that are part of the domino-like signaling pathway that work by phosphorylating proteins (add a small phosphate molecule) to change their activity. The Plk1 kinase plays an important role in mitosis of the cell that is replicating the cell causing the tumor to grow. You will recall that preventing mitosis was the job of the toxic taxane chemotherapy drugs. The gene for producing Plk1 is often up-regulated in cancer cells, which advances tumor growth. It also has other negative effects in that it promotes signaling of the androgen receptor. If that were not enough, it negatively regulates p53, the Guardian of the Genome, which is there to suppress tumors. It appears that inhibiting Plk1 with an inhibitor such as BI2536, while supplying Metformin, leads to a reduction in PCa growth, increased apoptosis of PCa cells, and reduces the progression from hormone sensitive to castrate resistant prostate cancer.

Let's first examine Metformin plus BI2536 experiments of human prostate cancer cells grown in the laboratory on plates with growth medium. This is the standard kind of test tube experiment to investigate drugs that can halt growth. Several types of prostate cancer cells were studied. **Figure 10-1** shows the number of colonies that grew under different conditions for two such PCa cell lines, LNCaP and C4-2. The LNCaP cell line is hormone sensitive and C4-2 is castrate resistant. C4-2 comes from LNCaP upon progression. Each plate was seeded initially with 1,000 cells

168

spread over the plate. One cannot see a single cell with the naked eye, but the cells will grow into colonies and when the colony becomes large enough, they becomes visible. The top panel shows the growth of LNCaP cells without Metformin or BI2536 (the control), and with each drug separately and in combination. One sees the power of the

Figure 10-1: Growth in a cell medium of Prostate Cancer cells (LNCaP top, C4-2 bottom) without drugs (control), or with Metformin or BI2536 alone, or in combination. All plates start with 1,000 cancer cells, which grow into visible colonies. (Data from C Shao et al., Journal of Biological Chemistry 290(4), 2024 (2015).)

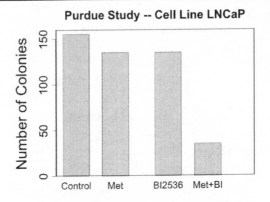

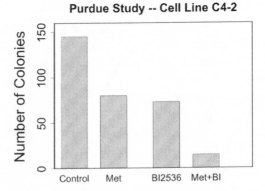

combination. Growth is severely halted when Metformin and BI2536 are used in combination. In the castrate resistant cell line C4-2, we see that either Metformin or BI2536 alone reduces colony formation by about half, but in combination (Met+BI) the growth is dramatically reduced.

p-53 is a tumor suppressor, and can cause cancer cells to undergo apoptosis (programmed death). The fact that cancer cells can avoid apoptosis is one of the hideous qualities of cancer. One can check if a cell is preparing for apoptosis by checking the cell for a specific enzyme, cleaved poly(ADP-ribose) polymerase, or c-PARP. To check for c-PARP, experimenters lyse the cells, purify the contents, and then run the cell's proteins through a protein electrophoresis gel in an electric field (SDS-PAGE technique) to separate proteins into bands of different length. The proteins in the gel are then transferred to a second gel that further identifies them by antibodies (Western blotting). This information allows us to determine if our cells are expressing c-PARP. If they are, celebrate. That means the cell is preparing to undergo cell death; a very welcomed event for a PCa cell. What is found is that in LNCaP and C4-2 cells the met+BI2536 combination produced more c-PARP than either drug does alone. Further good news is that normal prostate cells (not cancerous) did not produce c-PARP appreciably when exposed to either drug or in combination. Unfortunately this is also true of a cell line PC3 that was cancerous but was aberrant in that it did not express p53. Apparently we need p53, Guardian of the Genome, to be present for Metformin and BI2536 to be effective. Related to this, it is found that the dosage of Metformin needed to have antitumor activity is reduced with BI2536.

Positive results were also found in experiments with mice. Five million PCa cells were infused into the flanks of individual mice. After 12 days the mice were castrated. Tumor progression was followed for 75 days. Again there were 4 groups—a control (no Metformin or BI2536), a Metformin group, a BI2536 group, and a combination (Met+BI2536) group. Dosages of BI2536 (twice per week)

170

and Metformin were both 5mg/kg, which in human equivalents amounts to 500mg for a 100kg (220 lb) man. At the end of the trial, the tumor weights of the Metformin (alone) and BI2536 (alone) were about one-half that of the control group. Again synergy of the two drugs is found for the combination-treated mice with a tumor volume of about 11% of the control group.

There have been some Phase-I and -II clinical trials of BI2523 alone, performed on patients with recurrent or metastatic solid tumors (e.g. NCT00526149). They involve intravenous dosages of say 60 mg on days 1, 2, and 3, then repeat every 3 weeks, or 100mg on days 1 and 8, then repeat every 3 weeks. The BI2536 dosage in humans is significantly less (per kg body weight) than that what was given to mice. Neutropenia (low white blood cell count) can result in humans, and increases rapidly with dosage.

BI2536 was the first discovered Plk1-inhibitor discovered, and it may not be the best. Another inhibitor, BI6727 (Volasertib), may be better suited. However, all of this is experimental and the jury is out on just about all of this. The results presented here give us a preliminary peek as to what might develop as a useful therapy in the future.

References

On the Origin of Cancer Cells, Otto Warburg, Science 123 (3191). 309-314 (1959).

The effects of nonspecific HIF1a inhibitors on development of castrate resistance and metastases in prostate cancer, WKB Ranasinghe, S Sengupta, S Williams, M Chang, A Shulkes, DM Bolton, G Baldwin and O Patel, Cancer Medicine 3(2): 245–251 (2014).

Metformin and Prostate Cancer: Reduced Development of Castration-resistant Disease and Prostate Cancer Mortality, DE Spratt, C Zhang, ZS Zumsteg, X Pei, Z Zhang, and MJ Zelefsky, European Urology 63, 709-716 (2013).

Letter to the Editor Re: DE Spratt, C Zhang, ZS Zumsteg, X Pei, Z Zhang, MJ Zelefsky, Metformin and Prostate Cancer: Reduced Development of Castration-resistant Disease and Prostate Cancer

Mortality, L Bensimon, S Suissaa, L Azoulay, European Urology, 64, e28 (2013).

Letter to the Editor, Reply to L Bensimon, S Suissa, and L Azoulay's Letter to the Editor re: DE Spratt, C Zhang, ZS Zumsteg, X Pei, Z Zhang, MJ Zelefsky, Metformin and Prostate Cancer: Reduced Development of Castration-resistant Disease and Prostate Cancer Mortality, DE Spratt, Z Zhang and MJ Zelefsky, European Urology, 64, e29-e30 (2013).

Combination statin/metformin and prostate cancer specific mortality: A population-based study. GL Lu-Yao, Y Lin, D Moore, J Graff, A Stroup, K McGuigan, S Crystal, S Amin, K Demissie, and RS DiPaola, Journal of Clinical Oncology 33, suppl; abstr 5018 (2015).

Metformin in Chemotherapy-naive Castration-resistant Prostate Cancer: A Multicenter Phase 2 Trial (SAKK 08/09), C Rothermundt, S Hayoz, AJ Templeton, R Winterhalder, RT Strebel, D Bartschi, M Pollak, L Lui, K Endt, R Schiess, JH Ruschoff, R Cathomas, S Gillessen, European Urology 66, 468-474 (2014).

Metformin does not predict for prostate cancer diagnosis, grade, or volume of disease after transperineal template-guided mapping biopsy, GS Merrick, A Bennett, T Couture, WM Butler, RW Galbreath, and E Adamovich, American Journal of Clinical Oncology, Jan. 8 (2015).

Effect of metformin on prostate cancer outcomes after radical prostatectomy D Kaushik, RJ Karnes, MS Eisenberg, LJ Rangel, RE Carlson, EJ Bergstralh, Urologic Oncology: Seminars and Original Investigations 32, 43.e1–43.e7 (2014).

Inhibition of Polo-like Kinase 1 (Plk1) Enhances the Antineoplastic Activity of Metformin in Prostate Cancer, C Shao, N Ahmad, K Hodges, S Kuang, T Ratliff, and X Liu, Journal of Biological Chemistry, 290(4), 2024-2033 (2015).

Chapter 11

How The Body Fights Trouble— Introduction to Immunotherapy

I like the dreams of the future better than the history of the past. Thomas Jefferson

The immune system is a force to be reckoned with— that is if you are a foreign pathogen such as a bacterium or virus. A simple skin cut could lead to your death if your immune system were not there to save you. It is a complex system yet it takes only a small part of the genes in our DNA to construct it. But those genes produce powerful protection. Additionally, as we learn how to control and manipulate the immune system, new avenues for cancer therapy become possible. An informal comment of the Society for Immunotherapy of Cancer (SITC) is "CURE...Yeah We Said It!" Understanding the immune system opens the door to understanding the future of PCa therapy, perhaps leading to a cure in time.

We are interested in cancer immunotherapy and specifically applied to prostate cancer. This therapeutic avenue has great potential and promise but it is still largely a dream. We need new avenues of therapy for advanced prostate cancer to complement the well-trodden avenues of hormone therapy, chemotherapy, and radiation as they offer little in the form of a cure. The well-trodden avenues can even oppose immunotherapy—for example, chemotherapy deadens a patient's immune response. Thomas Jefferson has it right—let's dream of a better future then follow history. His dreaming brought us the great American political experiment, while cancer immunotherapy is an experiment that someday may finally control cancer. The journal "*Science,*" the premier journal for research scientists in the United States, named immunotherapy the breakthrough of 2013.

Cancer immunotherapy has at least three frontiers. They are adoptive T-cell therapy, anticancer vaccines, and immune checkpoint inhibitors. Adoptive T-cell therapy involves activating T-cells outside the patient, perhaps with modified genes, and infusing them back into the patient. Anticancer vaccines are vaccines not necessarily to prevent cancer but rather to produce an immune response that attacks the already present cancer. Finally, immune checkpoint inhibitors are antibodies that aid the patient's immune system by "taking its foot off the breaks" that prevent the immune system from being fully activated. All of these therapies have shown promising results in specific cancers and are viable candidates for prostate cancer.

Our Lewis-and-Clark-like journey is now going to take us through some white water—Immunology. We will try to calm the waters and in this chapter focus only on key concepts to help navigate the immunology frontiers of future chapters. The mission is to offer enough up-front information so that following chapters make some sense. Our agenda focuses on the major components used in prostate cancer immunotherapy—antigens, cytotoxic T-cells (Tc-cells), and dendritic cells. These are the "must-understand" components and will be described below.

Table 11-1. The players	
Proteins	
Antigens	A section or piece of protein that the immune system recognizes.
Antibodies	A complex of proteins with a "magnetic-like" attraction to a very specific antigen.
Membrane receptors	Much like an antibody, it is attracted to an antigen but is not free floating but is on the surface of cells.
Major Histocompatibility Complexes(MHC-I &II)	Cells digest foreign (cancerous) proteins into antigens, and then present them on their surface

	attached to MHC molecules.
Clusters of differentiation (CD-x)	Protein complexes on the surface of cells. Cells display specific CD's (e.g. CD-4 or CD-8) on their surface. These can be probed by antibodies to help us identify the cell's differentiation (i.e. the type of cell it is).
Cells	
Phagocytes	Phage=eat, cyte=cell. Cells that eat (digest) other cells to eliminate them. Macrophage (big eater) is a key example.
Dendritic Cells	Cells that digest foreign (cancerous) antigens and display them on MHC complexes on their surface to activate T-cells.
Lymphocytes	A class of immune cells that spend much time in lymph nodes. They include T-cells, B-cells, and NK-cells.
Cytotoxic T-cells (Tc)	T-cells programmed to attack cells that display a foreign (for example cancerous) antigen.
Other T cells	T helper (Th), regulatory (Treg)
B cells	Present antigens to T-cells, and flood the blood stream with antibodies targeted toward neutralizing pathogens.
Plasma cells	Mature B-cells that are factories for antigens to be spread throughout the body.
Natural Killer (NK) cells.	A very aggressive T-cell that skips some of the precautionary steps T-cells normally take.

Describing the function of the immune system will be confusing if we do not understand the names of the major players and what they do. (See **Table 11-1.**) This is so you can organize them in our minds. But they all play as a team and it is as a team that the true synergy of the players becomes apparent.

The immune system contains two layers, the innate immune system and the adaptive immune system. In a military analogy the innate system contains the Ground Forces while the adaptive system are the Special Forces. The innate system is a generalist, existing from the beginning, and does not learn. It offers the first layer of protection against invaders and includes defenses that are nonspecific. This includes defenses like mucosal linings in the nose and destructive enzymes in tears, sweat, or saliva. It also includes macrophages and neutrophils, cells that literally eat foreign and dead cells.

In contrast, the adaptive immune system is very specific. It learns as it goes and takes time (several days to weeks) to respond. The time it takes to get over the flu is an example of your adaptive immune system at work. The response time depends what it has already learned. Precious activations provide memory and rapid response times. The adaptive system attacks invaders that make it past the innate system and are recognized as not being part of the patient, thus "non-self." A troubling feature of cancer cells is that they are "self-cells" and the adaptive immune system must recognize them as targets. Cancer cells that thrive are those that have rid themselves of potential antigens or hiding themselves undercover in a stealthy environment—they are hidden from the immune system. The adaptive immune system will be the system that concerns us most in cancer immunotherapy. The big players of the adaptive immune system are T-cells and B-cells. These, along with natural killer (NK) cells, are in the class of white blood cells called lymphocytes, since they spend much of their time in lymph nodes. Lymphocytes are a type of white blood cell. White blood cells originate from stem cells in bone marrow, and find their way inside tissue and the region around cells. Lymphocytes interact with the thymus, thyroid and spleen.

The active ingredients of most immunotherapy protocols are T-cells. The immunotherapy may not directly manipulate T-cells, but whatever they do manipulate has the end purpose of getting T-cells, specifically cytotoxic T-cells, to act by attacking cancer cells.

The immune system is fine tuned to attack foreign pathogens, which includes bacteria and viruses. The system is first engaged when it encounters a bit of foreign protein called an antigen. It purposely is refined so as not to become engaged with self-proteins. This distinction between foreign- and self-proteins becomes blurred with cancer—cancer cells are aberrant self-cells, so their proteins are largely "self." Mutations and other aberrants make them non-self.

Evolution took a long time to develop the immune system, but we need to understand it quickly. We will go through each of the major pieces one at a time so that we can later put the whole picture together. T-cells are just part of a large team. We have to know something about all the players in order to understand how the game is played. This means understanding at some levels what all the players on a baseball team do, and not just know about the batter.

Before we begin, take a look at **Figure 11-1**. It shows a cartoon of a cell with its outer membrane and its nucleus inside housing the DNA. The membrane is home to proteins, and a couple of them are shown; a membrane receptor and a type-2 major histocompatibility complex that is presenting an antigen to the outside world.

Proteins Of Immunology

Proteins are what your DNA codes for. They are a linked chain of amino acids, usually hundreds of them, but they are not just simply long molecules. Tar is a long molecule but that does make it more powerful than octane. Proteins are far more amazing than just long molecules. They are tiny machines, performing specific tasks. They do this by folding up in a reproducible fashion and grabbing, pinching, cutting, filtering or holding other molecules or

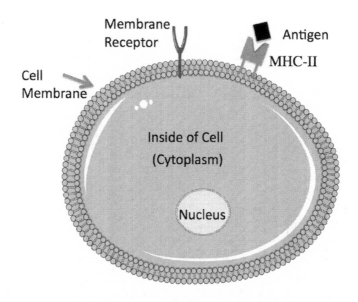

Figure 11-1. A cartoon of a cell showing its outer cell membrane, the cytoplasm and the nucleus. The membrane is home to many proteins. Shown are a membrane receptor and an MHC-II complex presenting an antigen.

proteins. If you say "who cares," then you will likely never understand how that pill you take works. There are tens of thousands of proteins. Thankfully we will be only looking at those of critical importance in the immune system. More information on proteins is given in the opening of Chapter 6, which gives some detail to the amino acids that compose the protein chain. The androgen receptor (Figure 3.1) and the CYP17A1 enzyme (Figure 5.3) give examples of protein chains and how they fold up.

178

Antigen

If there is anything you take away from this chapter, it is the concept of an antigen. Its importance comes from it being the identification tag that the immune system uses to identify a "wanted" character. Antigens are like the stripes on a prisoner's uniform that identifies its occupant as wanted and perhaps dangerous immediately after their prison bust.

Antigens are molecules that the immune system recognizes. If they are strong enough to produce an immune response they are immunogens. Often the distinction is not made between an antigen and an immunogen, so neither will we. An antigen is a portion of a protein, and usually of a foreign protein such as a bacterium. Being foreign, the body produces an immune response to attack the cell that is carrying it. An antigen is not a specific protein, but is a generic term referring to any protein, or portion of a protein that induces an immune response. The portions of a protein that a immune system player recognizes are called epitopes. There may be many epitopes on a single protein; one protein may have many antigens on it. Think of the body as a protein, the finger as an antigen, and the spot you place your ring on that finger as an epitope. The term antigen is so general that an antigen does not actually have to be protein, but for our purposes it will be. An antigen can also be nucleic acids (DNA or RNA) or foreign carbohydrates. We will be accurate to think of antigens as proteins or protein fragments from a foreign bit of material, and that the immune system can respond to. This really is the important idea.

Responding to the antigen is the goal. The idea is that the antigen comes from an invader such as a bacterial cell or a virus. And when the immune system encounters it, the immune system is activated and ultimately attacks cells that carry the antigen. The body knows that it is foreign because it has been trained early in life to know "self," that is proteins that it makes itself. We have a lot of proteins but it is a pittance compared to what is possible. Just a string of 10 amino-acids can be made 20^{10} different ways, since each spot along the string can be made of one of 20 different amino acids. That's one hundred thousand billion possibilities just for a string of 10. Proteins are hundreds or thousands long. There is no need to give the numbers—they are staggering.

Antibodies (and membrane receptors)

Say you have an antigen consisting of a foreign protein fragment. How does the immune system detect it? That is the role of antibodies. Antibodies are able to bind to very specific antigens. They are like tailor made magnets that are attracted to not just any piece of protein, but specific pieces containing a specific sequence and structure of amino acids. Although the way they are constructed and how they function is complex, their functional goal is simple—to find a very specific antigen out of millions (actually far more than that) of possibilities, and attach itself to it—this marks it for an action, such as destruction.

Antibodies are themselves constructed of proteins, a

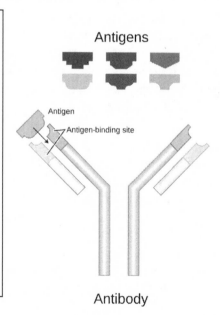

Figure 11-2. (Bottom) An antigen binding to the binding site of a Y-shaped antibody protein. (Top) The top shows several antigens, but only one antigen will bind to that specific antibody. (After Wikipedia, antibodies)

class of proteins called immunoglobulins. An antibody contains four proteins aggregated together and are depicted in illustrations as a "Y," shown in **Figure 11-2**. The four proteins in this aggregate, 2 long ones called the heavy chains and 2 small ones called the light chains, produce this general shape. The top part of the Y is the "business end" and is the portion that is specific to adhere to an antigen. Either side of the two top parts of the Y will grasp the antigen which is a very specific portion of the foreign protein (an epitope of the antigen). Since there are so many possible antigens, there needs to be a correspondingly large number of antibodies. The two-chain motif increases the number of specific antibodies that can bind to specific antigens. Each antibody is looking for a specific invader such as what occurs during an infection. Antibodies find that needle in a haystack. Of course, the end game is to produce a cascade of events signaling an immune response to destroy cells carrying that antigen. Antibodies are manufactured by B-cell lymphocytes, which mature in bone marrow.

Membrane receptors are similar to antibodies but are not free-floating like antibodies. They are attached to the cell membrane and are used to signal the cell when an antigen becomes attached to the receptor. Although similar to antibodies, membrane receptors have a different overall structure. The membrane receptor that will be particularly important is the T-cell receptor, or TCR. This tells the T-cell that it has found an "enemy combatant." Membrane receptors are different from free-floating receptors like the androgen receptor. The androgen receptor is a completely different component and is not part of the immune system, but rather a factor for gene expression. It is called a receptor because it receives androgen.

MHC

The next component is a matchmaker—that is to present the antigen to an antibody or receptor. That is the role of a protein complex called the major histocompatibility complex (MHC). There are two classes of MHC protein complexes, denoted MHC-I and MHC-II. These proteins reside on the surface of cells projecting out to the outside world. They are attached to the cell with one foot (MHC-I) or two feet (MHC-II). MHC-II exists on the surface of an antigen presenting cells (dendritic cells, see below), on B-cells and macrophages. MHC-I exists on the surface of any nucleated cell, meaning a cell with a nucleus containing DNA. (Almost all cells are nucleated. Red blood cells are an important example of a non-nucleated cell.)

What MHCs do is amazing. Their job is to present antigens from inside the cell to antibodies/receptors on the outside. It solves the "inside-outside" problem of showing some unusual or bad elements deep within the cell to the outside world where antibodies/receptors can "read" them. The MHC molecules may also act as a white flag of peace. The antigen is the enemy, and the MHC tells the offense that the cell is not an offender, but merely a messenger that these antigens are lurking elsewhere. Macrophage ingests antigen, digests it partially, and displays it on its surface. Pieces are displayed on MHC. Dendritic cells, a main player in our story, also present antigens on MHCs on their surface.

Clusters of Differentiation (CD)

Cells express unique clusters of proteins on their surface, that is on the cell membrane lipid layer. There is a very large class of these proteins, actually protein complexes as they are made generally of more than one protein, called Clusters of Differentiation, or CD for short. Cells initially are derived from stem cells that can produce many different kinds of cell. The process of a cell being produced that is very specific is called differentiation. For example, lymphoidal cells start from a hematapoetic stem cell source, and that source produces either a B-cell, a T-cell, or a natural killer (NK) cell. The clusters of differentiation have names like CD1, CD2, ... and are named in the order of their discovery.

We care about CDs for two reasons. First, we can identify the type of cell it is by what CDs it is expressing. It is difficult to determine the identity of a cell just by looking at it, as often they are odd shapes and different types are mixed togehter. B-cells express CD-19, cytotoxic T-cells express CD-8, and T-helper cells express CD-4. We can tell which CD a cell has, and hence what kind of cell it is, by adding to the cell dish engineered antibodies that fluoresce (glow in light) by sticking to a specific CD.

The second reason is CDs perform function. In the context of immunology, they often are attachment points for one cell to attach, by a receptor, to another.

Cells

Before describing key cells of the immune system, it is useful to reflect on the clonal selection hypothesis to see what the rules of engagement are.

Clonal Selection Hypothesis

The clonal selection hypothesis forms the foundation of understanding the workings of the immune system. It is a set of "laws" that govern behavior of the immune system's lymphocytes. Underlying the hypothesis is that lymphocytes (B-, T-, and NK-cells) bind to antigens with high affinity by using a receptor on the surface of the lymphocycte, and that when activated, lymphocyctes reproduce to increase the number of lymphocyte cells that can attack the pathogen.

A. **One target:** Lymphocytes have a receptor on their surface that is specific for one and only one antigen. There may be a large number (thousands) of these specific receptors on the lymphocyte surface.

B. **Finding results in activation:** The lymphocyte receptor will bind strongly to its target antigen when it is found, and causes the lymphocyte to be activated.

C. **Activation produces identical copies:** An activated lymphocyte will produce replicas to help destroy pathogens, and the replicas have receptors that target the same antigen as the parent.

D. **Self-targeting cells are filtered out:** Developing lymphocyte cells are removed early if they have receptors that target self-molecules. The mature immune system should only have non-self targetting lymphocyctes.

The one target law states that mature lymphocytes are hunting for just one type of prey. It is like they have the "Wanted Poster" in their pocket with just one wanted target. It is not like a cop on the beat that may have access to a tall pile of wanted posters. This is very different from what you may have thought that there are many different kinds of receptors on the surface of a lymphocyte, and binding any one of them causes activation. A consequence of the one target rule is that one needs a vary large variety of lymphocytes. It is only by "finding" that produces identical copies that results in many copies of that particular receptor carrying lymphocyte. These progeny are called effector cells—they are ready to hunt for pathogens and effect an immune response. The identical-copies-law explains why it takes time to get over a virus infection (the specific population must build up from an initially small number), and why reinfection at a later date is likely to not even be noticed (many lymphocytes for that pathogen are now available to fight and neutralize the infection quickly). The filtering of lymphocytes of self-targeting receptors keeps the immune system from attacking its host. This filtering is done in the thymus for T-cells and in bone marrow for B-cells. It is performed on immature cells, and once it is done, it is irreversible. Those cells are no longer in the pool and the phenomenon is clonal deletion.

Phagocytes
Phagocytes translate to (phage) eater (cytes) cells. One of the most important in this class are macrophages, which are a type of leukocyte (white blood cell). Their name macrophage tells it all—macro (large) + phage (eater). These are very large cells that clean up debris and pathogens. They are like vacuum cleaners sucking up harmful agents in our blood and tissue, including dead tissue. They are multifunctional, also acting as the trigger for an immune

response. Antigens are taken in by the macrophages and digested. They are called an antigen presenting cell, or APC. APCs are what activate the immune system, as the immune system does not respond to antigens directly, but by having them presented to them on a "silver platter," the silver platter is an MHC molecule. Macrophages present pieces of proteins (antigens) on their surface. They do this by presenting the antigen at the end of the MHC-II protein sticking out the macrophage's surface. It is an alert to the rest of body that it has found something of concern. This is the trigger ready to be pulled by other agents of the immune system. In summary: Macrophage ingests antigen, digests it partially, and display antigens on its surface on an MHC-II.

Dendritic Cells

Another antigen presenting cell is a dendritic cell (DC). This cell has a special place in our hearts because it forms the foundation for many of the cancer vaccine immunotherapies to be discussed in later chapters such as Sipuleucel-T (Provenge).
Dendritic cells are part of the innate immune system, but they "talk" to T-cells which are part of the adaptive immune system. Being part of the innate system means that they are fairly indiscriminant. They are searching for any type of pathogen through receptors on their surface or they "nibble" small portions of suspect cells. This causes the DCs to mature, and then after internalizing the antigen and chopping it up into small antigen pieces, they present the antigens on their surface through an MHC-II complex. This is the event Tc-cells have been hunting for. The Tc-cells bind onto the antigen/MHC-II complex and are stimulated into activation.

T-cells

The entire immune system is a complex system, but T-cells are particularly difficult to get straight as to what they do, as they have different "flavors" and perform several functions. The most important variety for prostate immunotherapy is cytotoxic T-cells (Tc-cells). More generally, T-cells are developed in the thymus gland (hence T) in our upper chest between the lungs. T-cells circulate continuously throughout the body searching for targets.

There are two general varieties of T-cells; cytotoxic T-cells (Tc cells) and helper T-cells (Th cells). Th cells also have subclasses Th1, Th2, Th17 and Treg (regulatory) cells. Each of these varieties and subclasses perform different functions. A feature that distinguishes Tc cells from Th cells is that Tc cells present CD8 on their surface (hence are also called CD8$^+$ cells), while Th cells are CD4$^+$.

The most important point about Tc-cells is that they bind to an antigen presented to them on an MHC—antigens by themselves are not enough. The binding of the antigen/MHC-complex and the T-cell occurs via the Tc-cell receptor (TCR), and is the initiating event in the production of an immune response. The antigen on the MHC is on the surface of an antigen-presenting cell (APC). Often dendritic cells are used as APCs in prostate cancer immunotherapy, but let us not forget other APCs such as macrophages. The existence of an APC is an important concept in the development of immunotherapy. The claw on the Tc-cell that adheres to the MHC-antigen is the T-cell receptor (TCR). The TCR is similar to an antibody. It has a constant region and a variable region and it is designed by nature to stick to one antigen. Each Tc-cell has many of the same Tc-cell receptors on its surface.

When presented with the antigen by an APC, the T-cell jumps into action. It is only the APC and T-cell combination that produce a response—like a car needs a driver. The binding causes the T-cell to proliferate and to seek out foreign or tumor-like antigens on cells. The proliferation of these specific cytotoxic T-cells takes a few days. A virus infected person does not get well immediately, but it takes time for the T-cells to accumulate and do their job. The job of these activated mature cytotoxic T-cells is to kill an infected cell that presents the specific antigen that it recognizes. Like the macrophages, an infected cell presents the antigen but now on an MHC-I protein.

The nickname of cytotoxic T-cells is killer T-cells. They get their name by attaching to the antigen-class I MHC complex on the infected cell and releasing a protein (perforin) that drills holes into the cell releasing its contents—a sort of bleeding to death. After the T-cells have done their job they die off. But a few remain and become cytotoxic memory cells. If the person is exposed a second time to the pathogen, the immune system is ready to pounce on it. The killer T-cells do their job much more quickly the second time around, and the person may not even know they were infected.

We now give a summary of the process, imagining a cell that is infected by a virus. Although we are interested in tumor cells, the generic principles are similar.

1. Foreign Antigen. An infected cell has a foreign antigen on its surface.

2. Macrophage (APC). Gobbles up the infected cell.

3. APC MHC-II. Presents antigen of the infected cell on an MHC-II protein on its surface.

4. T-cell binds. A Tc-Cell, with the proper T-cell receptor (TCR) binds to the antigen.

5. Signaling. The binding causes a signaling to occur by molecules (interleukins).

6. T-cell mature and grow. Signaling causes T-cells to reproduce and mature (killer Tc).

7. Infected cell+MHC-I+antigen. An infected cell has antigen on its surface.

8. Killer T-cell binds. The mature Tc-cell (Killer T-cell) binds to the MHC-I/antigen.

9. Infected cell dead. Killer Tc emits perforin (perforates the cell), and infected cell dies.

That is a lot of steps and seems overly complex. But the immune system must be complex to have checks and balances so that it does not destroy you.

B cells

The most important function of B cells is to produce antibodies that are specific to an offending antigen.

Antibodies are fluid soluble and are good for attacking free floating pathogens like bacteria. The offending target-antigen usually is from a virus or bacterium, but in our case we want it to be from a cancer cell. The purpose of producing antibodies is that they can diffuse around in fluid and eventually attach themselves to distant target-antigens on cells, viruses, or bacterium. This attachment marks them for destruction by other immune system components.

B-cells exist in the humoral (fluid) immune system such as blood. The products of B-cells, antibodies (immunoglobulins), are also released into the humoral system. B-cells are matured in bone marrow (B for Bone) and when matured, they have different functions. They act as hunters—hunters seeking a very specific prey. On their surface are immunoglobulins. They bind very specific portions of very specific antigens. When they find an antigen that binds to their antibody, they act somewhat like macrophages. They engulf the antigen and its attachments, and partially digest it and then display the antigen on its surface on MHC proteins.

The end game here is to produce more antibodies and more B cells, both of which are specific to only this antigen. To do this it needs help. That is supplied by helper T-cells (Th-cells). Mature helper T-cells have already encountered the same antigen through the macrophage, so it is being signaled to help this particular B-cell. When it binds to the B-cell, it releases signaling (interleukin) molecules. These molecules signal back to the B cell that it should grow and proliferate, producing B cells with the same surface immunoglobulins. The army against the offending antigen is growing.

Interleukin molecules signal the B cell to not only multiply but to also make drastic changes (differentiate) as they reproduce. The change for most is to produce another kind of cell, a Plasma cell. The cell loses its surface antibodies, and begins to secrete antibodies into the blood. The secreted antibodies are the same antibodies that target the offending antigen. These secreted antibodies are now ready to do their job. In large numbers, they float around and bind to antigens when they are encountered. Foresters mark trees for harvest by leaving a mark on the trunk. The bound antibody on the antigen is the death mark for what carries the antigen. Another eating cell of the immune system, a phagocyte, recognizes the death mark and devours the cell (phagocytosis).

There is another mechanism that comes into play with "death marked" components, the complement immune system. The complement immune system contains a couple dozen or so proteins in blood plasma that lyse (cut up) cells, or attracts phagocytes (the eater cells) to act on a marked cell. A cut of the skin produces redness and swelling produced by the complement system as it surrounds the area and recruits phagocytes into the area.

Not all B cells reproduce into plasma cells. Another change that occurs for some of the B cells is that they go into reserve, as memory B cells. These are ready to jump into action quickly in case the same antigen appears at a later date.

Molecules (some of which are actually proteins)

Molecules play an important role to signal and change the behavior of cells, and in particular immune cells. Your patience has already been tried if you made it to here, so I'll be brief and just list the major players and go into very slight detail with a couple of them. See **Table 11-2**.

Interleukins are signaling molecules between cells. Their name "between whites" reflects that their original function was thought only to be between leukocytes (white blood cells) of the immune system. Like many things in biochemistry, they multitask and signal other cells as well. Although they are listed here as a molecule, truth be told they too are proteins, and belong to a larger class of cell messenger molecules called **cytokines**. Interleukins have easy to remember names; IL1, IL2 and so on. The release of interleukins is partially responsible for inflammation that occurs during an immune response such as infection.

Table 11-2 The players: Molecules	
Cytokines	A general term for a class of signaling molecule that includes interleukins, interferon, colony stimulating factor, chemokines, tumor necrosis factor.
Interleukins	Signaling molecule that causes T-cell to become activated when attached to an APC.
Kinase	An enzyme that transfers a phosphate group onto a protein. This changes the behavior of the protein, and is used as a part of a signaling cascade in cells.
Interferon	Enhance immune response by signaling non-infected nearby cells of an imminent infection. Also they can interfere with tumor growth.
Chemokines	Signaling molecules that recruits immune cells to an infection site.
Tumor necrosis factor (TNF)	A protein that can produce apoptosis (cell death) of tumor cells. Also can stimulate immune cells.
Colony Stimulating Factors (CSF)	Proteins that stimulate the production of white blood cells. Often given with PCa immunotherapies, and in chemotherapy to fight resulting neutropenia (low white blood cell count).

Interleukins, and more generally cytokines, create a telegraph system between molecules that contain instructions for the receiving cell to act. The sending cell releases its messenger molecule and it docks onto a receptor for the receiving molecule of the receiving cell. Message received. This instructs the receiving cell to act. For our purposes, the prime example of interleukin signaling is that which occurs when the T-cell receptor of a T-cell binds to an MHC presented antigen on an antigen presenting cell. ILs are released by the APC to stimulate the T-cell to reproduce and develop and the T-cell releases its own ILs to signal other T-cells that an infection is present. Cancer cells fight the immune system. One way to do this is that cancer cells produce suppressive cytokines to turn off the immune response. Interleukins and cytokines produce a tug of war between stimulating and suppressing the immune system.

Kinases are molecules that transfer phosphate groups to other molecules in a process called phosphorylation. That sounds as dull as dishwater, but this step is a key step in stimulation of receptors and other molecules that push forward events to activate bigger players like cells. Some oncogenes like those that produce the RAS protein initiate a kinase cascade. RAS starts a domino-like series of kinase events to stimulate the cell to grow. If the RAS gene is mutated, it can produce uncontrolled growth leading to cancer—all becasue of runaway kinase activity.

The group of kinases of interest here are protein kinases, which are enzymes. They cut and mend bonds between atoms in a protein. The phosphate group that is cut and mended is (PO_4^{3-}). This group comes from ATP (Adenosine Triphosphate) which includes a tail of three (tri-) phosphate groups packed together. ATP is the energy molecule, a kind of biological fuel for the body. The packing of three phosphates costs energy to build, and energy is released when one phosphate is removed to form ADT (Adenosine Diphosphate). The enzymatic activity of the protein kinase can be written as, Protein + ATP → (Phosphorylated Protein) + ADP. The enzyme is not written, as it is the enabler—the means for the reaction to occur. The important result is to change a target protein into a phosphorylated protein, where the phosphorylated protein has different activity and binding properties than the starting protein.

References

"Biochemistry", 2nd Edition, D. Voet and J.G. Voet, John Wiley & Sons, pp 1207-1211 (1995).

The T-cell and Its Receptor, Philippa Marrack and John Kappler, Scientific American 254(2), 36-45 (1986).

Immuno Biology, The immune system in health and disease," CA Janeway, P Travers, M Walport, M Shlomchik, 5th Edition, Garland Publishing, (New York NY), 2001.

Chapter 12

The Trouble With Immune Checkpoints: CTLA-4 And PD-1

… suspending the brakes. Not so much harnessing the immune system, but unleashing it to attack whatever it was going to attack.
Jim Allison (on CTLA-4 checkpoint inhibitors)

Treatments Of Prostate Cancer With Immunology

There are those that say immunological treatments will never work, and there are those that feel it is the one true cure that we are looking for. Expeditions are like that. Lewis and Clark were told they would be killed by wooly mammoths if not by a thousand other hazards. But they made it. Will immunotherapy get us to our goal?

There has been great progress in treating some cancers like melanoma with immunotherapy. Melanoma cancer is replete with mutations, which although undesirable generally, actually helps with immunotherapy since it offers more immunogenic targets. But does this mean immunotherapy will be effective in prostate cancer? T-cells and antigens are key players in the immunological battle. T-cells circulate in the blood and antigens are the signal that a foreign entity is in residence. Prostate cancer has the desirable feature that it has unique antigens. One is called PSMA (prostate specific membrane antigen) and of course PSA (prostate specific antigen) is another. In patients with their prostate removed, there should be no PSA or very little PSMA. Presence of these specific cancer modified antigens means that prostate cancer cells have a bulls-eye target painted on them for T-cells to zero in on.

Immune Checkpoints

The immune system is highly regulated. Our bodies perform many jobs and resources are limited. It cannot afford to pour all its resources into fighting phantom infections. Much like waging a war, resources must be parceled out where they do the most good. There are Go signals and there are Stop signals. Immune checkpoints are **stop** signals, often referred to as putting the brakes on the immune response. An immune checkpoint inhibitor does what its name suggests: it inhibits the application of the brakes. The immune response can carry on forward and hopefully attack our target, cancer cells.   The hero of this story is the maverick Jim Allison, now at the U. Texas MD Anderson in Houston who had "the selfish desire to be the first person on the planet to know something." He found the CTLA-4 protein did not turn on the immune system as all thought, but rather halted it. CTLA-4 is the brake, not the accelerator. Confusing brakes with accelerators can be even more dangerous in biology than it is in automobiles.

There are two checkpoint inhibitors that are being used to fight cancer. They are CTLA-4 and PD-1; the names will be defined later. Foremost about this approach is that they work on the immune system and not on the tumor. This is certainly a different way of thinking about the problem— out of the box as they say. The general ideas are not new as they were very active in the 1970s era. But experiments in mice did not pan out as hoped; so much for that idea. Now we know far more about the immune system and immune checkpoints are a relatively new discovery.

In addition, we also now know that immunotherapy does not work quickly. The tumor grows before positive results are found. In experiments with mice, the mice may be dead before an immunotherapy can be shown to be effective. This delay in activity has consequences for patients. One is that immunotherapy is best when given early, allowing more time for the therapy to work. Another is that progression will likely continue after administration of an immunotherapy.

For PCa patients this immediately means that PSA levels will not go down immediately. Months may be needed.

The name "Cytotoxic T lymphocyte-associated antigen 4" (CTLA-4) spells out the basics of CTLA-4. It is an membrane antigen on the surface of our immune friend cytotoxic-T (Tc) cells. These are the cells that we are trying to coax into attacking PCa cells. But PCa cells are self-cells, which the immune system avoids, and cancer cells set up an inhibitory environment to dull or remove an immune response.

Cytotoxic T-cells become activated, then they are told to stop, becoming inhibited or deactivated. CTLA-4 is part of the Tc-cell's inhibitory pathway. To understand how the regulation of Tc-cells works, we need to understand both the activation and deactivation process.

The primary step in activation is when an antigen-presenting cell (APC), such as a macrophage or **dendritic cell**, presents an antigen to the T-cell. The antigen is a protein fragment from a virus, bacterium, or cancer cell. The T-cell binds to the APC and the T-cell is trained to be sensitive to that antigen, by its T-cell receptor. That antigen is its hunted prey. But it also needs another stimulus, just as we need two stimuli to get up in the morning (an alarm and a cup of Joe). Signal 1 is the antigen presentation. Signal 2 insures that the T-cell is communicating with a legitimate source. Signal 2 is a second binding event between CD28 receptors on the T-cell, and CD80 or CD86 (called B7 ligands) molecules on the APC. Notice that the tumor cell is not yet involved; only the "scent" of the tumor cell is involved through the antigen presented by the APC. When the T-cell receives both signals 1 and 2 it is activated and is programmed to look for a specific target, the presented antigen. It also can proliferate. Lt. Gerard now has his warrant and assembles his deputies to hunt down and arrest Dr. Richard Kimbel, "The Fugitive."

That is what is supposed to happen. But the immune system is regulated in many ways and CTLA-4 is one of those ways. CTLA-4 is an antibody and is in the same family as the CD28 antibody that binds the T-cell to the B7 ligands. Thus it too can bind to B7 and binds more strongly. The difference is that binding CTLA-4 to B7 does not produce signal 2, as does binding CD28 to B7. Normally the number of CTLA-4 antibodies on the surface is much smaller than the number of CD28 antibodies. So even though CTLA-4 is stronger, they have less of a chance to perform this important "mating" dance.

Figure 12-1 illustrates how T-cells are activated and the role of CD80-CD28 and CTLA-4.

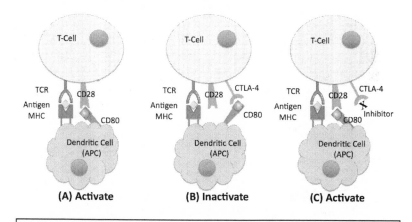

(A) Activate   (B) Inactivate   (C) Activate

Figure 12-1. How CTLA-4 inhibition works. ("A" panel) A dendritic cell (APC) with an antigen presented on its MHC binds to the T cell receptor (TCR) of the T cell. A second signal is needed to fully activate the T cell, and that is the binding of a CD80 (or CD86) to a CD28 on the T cell. ("B" Panel) The second signal causes the T-cell to express CTLA-4. But CTLA-4 binds better to CD80 (or CD86) than CD26, thus shutting down further activation. ("C" Panel) An antibody binds to CTLA-4 so that CD80 (or CD26) can again bind to CD20 to fully activate the T-cell so that it is hungry to attack tumors. (More details at A Vasaturo et al., Frontiers in Immunology 4(417), 1-14 (2013).)

The question is now, "How does CTLA-4 actually perform its regulation of the activation process of T-cells?"

The answer unfortunately is not entirely clear. But this is the wrong question to ask concerning a therapy. The important question is, "How to stop the regulation?" And that is by a CTLA-4 inhibitor. That is what this checkpoint inhibitory immunotherapy is all about—removing the regulation of CTLA-4 so that both signal 1 and signal 2 can occur and T-cells become activated and proliferate.

But let's at least look at some regulatory functions of CTLA-4 before moving on to the more important question of inhibition. The first was given above; the stronger binding CTLA-4 bullies the CD28 away from binding during activation. Other mechanisms are also at work. CTLA-4 alters the surface of the cell, the membrane layer, making a CD28-B7 connection more difficult. CTLA-4 also causes the T-cell to move around faster making contact of CD28 with B7 more difficult. Several things are going on with CTLA-4 binding, and we need to stop it.

Does It Work?

Anti-CTLA-4 in the form of Ipilimumab (Yervoy®), or Ipi for short, improves overall survival in metastatic melanoma with many (19-36%) having greater than a 4-year survival. It has been FDA approved for melanoma. Even though Ipi is FDA approved for melanoma, it was first investigated as a PCa immunotherapy. But the benefit of Ipi for PCa is far less clear.

There have been many clinical trials on PCa using anti-CTLA-4, but the jury is still out on its benefit. Most of the clinical trials were Phase I and Phase II, but there have been a couple Phase III trials. Most studies include only patients with mCRPC. Also, most combine Ipi with other therapies; GM-CSF (Granulocyte-Macrophage Colony Stimulating Factor), GVAX (Vaccine), Prostvac (Vaccine) + GM-CSF, Provenge (Vaccine), and other therapies like radiotherapy and chemotherapy (Docetaxel). Combining Ipi with other immunological therapies, like vaccines, makes sense in that Ipi aids the immune response if and only if an immune response occurs. But trials with combinations of therapies make it difficult to fully know the true benefit each therapy (such as Ipi) has produced in the combined therapy.

There is one study ongoing that compares just Ipilimumab vs. placebo (NCT01057810), "Phase 3 Study of Immunotherapy to Treat Advanced Prostate Cancer," but there are no reported results. So our information is very limited on answering the question "Does it work?"

In the combination therapies with other immuno-agents, there have been noticeable PSA responses and disease stabilization. In a GVAX + Ipi trial, 5 of 28 patients had a decline of PSA of greater than 50%. In a Phase II trial of Prostvac + GM-CSF plus Ipi on mCRPC, there were 6 patients that had already undergone chemotherapy and 24 who had not, for a total of 30 patients (NCT00124670). The patients who had undergone previous chemotherapy showed "no evidence of clinical benefit" with the combined Ipi therapy. Of the 30 patients in total, 14 showed some decline in PSA levels, but there was rarely reduction in tumor volume.

The results of a Phase I/II trial was published in 2013 which include those receiving Ipi alone versus those receiving Ipi + radiotherapy (*NCT00323882*). The concept is a good one, in that radiation will certainly kill cancer cells and release antibodies throughout the body. If the Ipi can help stimulate the immune system to respond to these antibodies, a very positive immune effect might occur on PCa cells at a distant site. Thus the two therapies work in synergy, a cooperative strategy underutilized in cancer therapy. The specific effect here is called the abscopal effect, also known as radiation driven immunotherapy. The abscopal effect (Latin for away from target) occurs when killing cancer cells in one place cause destruction of cancer in another place.

Fifty patients received the highest doses (10mg/kg) of Ipi: 16 Ipi only, 34 Ipi + radiotherapy. The results of all patients (radiotherapy or not) were these:
8 PSA declines of greater than 50% from 3-13 months, 1 complete response over 11 months, and 6 had stable disease

of duration 3-6 months. Let's do the math; 8+1+6=15 out of 50 patients, or 30% showed a definite benefit. But it's the one patient with the long-term complete PSA response that is the "head turning" success. Sadly, that is just 2% of the patients. It was not entirely clear what effect radiation had on those that received it. There were adverse effects. Adverse effects include diarrhea (over half of the patients), colitis, rash, pruritus (itching) and hepatitis One death related to the treatment occurred. I see the hopes for an abscopal effect dimming in light of this trial.

All in all, Ipi seems to have some positive effect on disease progression, but it is not showing outstanding results. That does not mean it never will. The right combination of variables, if one exists, is still not evident. I still hold out hope, especially in view of its effectiveness with other cancers like melanoma. But right now, it looks discouraging. I hope I'm wrong.

PD-1 Blockade Immunotherapy

Programmed Death 1 (PD-1) is a protein receptor on the surface of activated T-cells. Another protein acts as a ligand that binds to the PD-1 receptors. These ligands, PD-L1 or PD-L2, are on the surface of cancer cells. When T-cells encounter cancer cells, the PD-L1 protein binds to the PD-1 receptor on T-cells causing them to lose their function. This acts as a brake on the immune system. The PD-1 blockade immunotherapy inhibits the binding of PD-L1 to the PD-1 receptor, thus negating the braking effect.

To do this, we can block the attachment of PD-L1 to the PD-1 protein by instead using an antibody drug to bind to PD-1. The antibody used is a monoclonal antibody with the laboratory name BMS-936558, street name Nivolumab (Opdivo®).

This immunotherapy is referred to as a PD-1 blockade. The binding event of BMS-936558 does not brake the immune response like PD-L1 does. This allows the immune system to remain activated, thus allowing it to attack cancer cells.

A Phase I trial, concluded in 2012, tested this therapy on several cancers all in one study. The cancers were lung, kidney, colorectal, melanoma and castration resistant prostate cancer with a total of 296 patients. The CRPC sample was small, only 17 patients. The PD-1 blockade strategy found positive results in lung and kidney cancers and melanoma at a rate of 20-25%. The therapy has risks, and three deaths were noted from pulmonary disease.

What are its effects in prostate cancer? The Trial reports that there was no real effect on colorectal or prostate cancers. It is not clear why some cancers respond and others do not. It seems for prostate cancer that removing the brakes is not enough—automobiles immobilized by frozen transmissions are not mobilized by removing the brakes. We need an immune response to occur in the first place so that removing inhibitions have an effect. This trial had no other immunotherapy treatment, like a vaccine, to stimulate it. Perhaps with combination therapies, anti-PD-1 would be effective.

But there are other potential reasons why it failed. One being that PD-L1 is abundant in some cancer cells (like melanoma); it is not highly expressed on PCa cells. It is there, but perhaps not in high enough levels that it is a major factor in inhibiting T-cell attack. Inhibiting PD-L1 does little if PD-L1 is not truly doing much to inhibit T-cell attack. Again out Lewis and Clark expedition has led us into muddy waters. Research proceeds and as Yogi Berra famously said, "It ain't over till its over."

References

Phase I trial of targeted therapy with PSA-TRICOM vaccine (V) and ipilimumab (ipi) in patients (pts) with metastatic castration-resistant prostate cancer (mCRPC), M Mohebtash, RA Madan, PM Arlen, M Rauckhorst, KY Tsang, V Cereda, M Vergati, DJ Poole, WL Dahut, J Schlom, and JL Gulley, Journal of Clinical Oncology 27(15s), abstract 5144 (2009).

Overall survival (OS) analysis of a phase 1 trial of a vector-based vaccine (PSA-TRICOM) and ipilimumab (Ipi) in the treatment of metastatic castration-resistant prostate cancer (mCRPC), RA Madan, M Mohebtash, PM Arlen, M Vergati, SM Steinberg, KY Tsang, WL Dahut, J Schlom and JL Gulley, Journal of Clinical Oncology 28(15s) abstract 2550 (2010).

Ipilimumab alone or in combination with radiotherapy in metastatic castration-resistant prostate cancer: results from an open-label, multicenter phase I/II study, SF Slovin, CS Higano, O Hamid, S Tejwani, A Harzstark, JJ Alumkal, HI Scher, K Chin, P Gagnier, M B McHenry and TM Beer, Annals of Oncology 24, 1813–1821 (2013).

Clinical implications of co-inhibitory molecule expression in the tumor microenvironment for DC vaccination: a game of stop and go, A Vasaturo, S Di Blasio, DGA Peeters, CCH de Koning, JM de Vries, CG Figdor and SV Hato, Frontiers in Immunology 4(417), 1-14 (2013).

Progress in advanced Prostate Cancer, CN Sternberg, DP Petrylak, RA Madan, C Parker, 2014 ASCO meeting, ASCO.org/edbook.

Safety, Activity, and Immune Correlates of Anti–PD-1 Antibody in Cancer, SL Topalian, FS Hodi, JR Brahmer, SN Gettinger et al., New England Journal of Medicine 366, 2443- 2454 (2012).

Chapter 13

Vaccinating Trouble

Ralph Steinman created a revolution in immunology when he discovered a beautiful cell by just looking through a microscope. …. He showed that dendritic cells are critical for initiating the most important immune responses.
Michel C Nussenzweig, Nobel Prize lecture 2011.

Cancer vaccines are a great idea, but they have to do things just right to work effectively. And that is why there is no slam-dunk winner for prostate cancer yet, but the field is very active. There is some confusion about vaccines because there are two general categories of cancer vaccines. The first category is a *Preventative Vaccine*. These are closer to a conventional vaccine, such as for the flu, in that they reduce the risk or even prevent disease. Cancer vaccines in this category include human papilloma virus (HPV) for cervical cancer and hepatitis B (HEP-B) for liver cancer. The second category is a *Therapeutic Vaccine*. These are the immunotherapy vaccines that are the subject of this section and apply to prostate cancer.

There has been much press on therapeutic cancer vaccines for some types of cancer. In applications to prostate cancer, the results are encouraging, but so far they are not the killer-therapy that was hoped for. But they do have a place as they can slow down PCa progression and extend overall survival (a tiny bit). The can also be obscenely expensive. Therapeutic cancer vaccines are useful in combination with other therapies. Therapies that compromise the immune system, like chemotherapy, are not obvious partners to combine with. A puzzle is why some patients respond much better than others. Needed are biomarkers or indicators of which patients will have a large positive response.

Why is it so difficult to develop a therapeutic vaccine that works? The first reason is that your body has tolerated the cancer cells for some time before they are ever treated with a vaccine. The antigens in the tumor have already been presented to your immune system, but your immune system has failed to act, at least with sufficient effort to destroy the tumor. The second is that the cancer cells have developed their own microenvironment in which they live, and form a kind of moat. Biochemicals are secreted to enhance the survival of the tumor and thwart the immune response.

There are several vaccine therapies. Most of the discussion will be on Sipuleucel-T and Prostvac. They use two different agents to deliver immunotherapy; dendritic cells in one case and viruses in the other. The remaining therapies are variations, sometime very important variations, of these themes. The other important variable is the antigen being used to elicit an immune response. **Table 13-1** summarizes where we are going.

Table 13-1: Vaccine Therapy	Active agent	Tumor associated antigen
Sipuleucel-T (Provenge)	Patient's dendritic cells activate T-cells.	Prostatic acid phosphatase (PAP).
Prostvac	Engineered viruses	PSA antigen.
DCVAC	Patient's dendritic cells activate T-cells.	Antigens within whole LNCaP cells.
Others (DCVax, GVAX, BPX-201)	Patient's dendritic cells activate T-cells.	LNCaP cells, PSA, PSMA

Sipuleucel-T (Provenge)

The historically most important example for a prostate cancer vaccine is Sipuleucel-T (Sip-T). Sip-T, earlier known as APC8015, is an active immunotherapy in which T-cells of the patient are the agent that attacks the cancer tumor. But nothing is done to alter them. The therapy comes about by conditioning the patient's dendritic cells that present antigens to the T-cells. Recall that the process of activating T-cells starts with an antigen. Antigens do not directly activate T-cells but rather first must be internalized by another type of cell, an antigen-presenting cell (APC). There are different types of APCs, and the cells used in Sip-T are dendritic cells. An APC takes up the antigen and then presents it on a kind of silver platter to the T cell. The "silver platter" is an MHC-II (Major Histocompatibility Complex - 2) protein on the surface of the APC. Once presented, the T-cell binds to it and becomes activated. This is the trigger that sets off the destruction of the tumor.

The hero in the discovery of ideas that led to methods of vaccination like Sip-T is Ralph Steinman of Rockefeller University. What Steinman did was discover dendritic cells in 1973 and determined their role in the immune system. Dendritic cells are part of the innate immune system, but by presenting antibodies to T-cells, they activate the adaptive immune system. They play on both teams. Steinman received the Nobel Prize in Medicine in 2011. Curiously he died just a few days before the award was announced. The Nobel Prize committee did not know of his death when they announced the award, and were faced with a problem. Nobel Prizes can only be awarded to living persons. The rules allow the prize to be kept by the family if the recipient dies between the announcement and the award ceremony. That is not quite the case here, but common sense prevailed and the Prize was awarded posthumously. Michel Nussenzweig gave the Nobel Prize lecture at the award ceremony. The cause of Steinman's death was cancer—pancreatic cancer. This is a deadly form of cancer, yet he survived for four years with a treatment of his own design. The details of that treatment are not known.

Sip-T is not a drug, but a personalized procedure performed individually for each patient. One may hype it as a living drug. The destruction of cancer cells is performed by the patient's own immune system. The treatment helps to activate that system. Blood is taken from the patient and the white blood cells extracted by a leukapheresis technique. The sample is shipped to a laboratory for processing. There are three treatments, each separated by two weeks. So the whole affair lasts just four weeks. But timing is critical since it must be shipped back and forth between the patient's treatment center and the external laboratory with little delay. Mine was shipped to Georgia and I live in Arizona.

Centrifuges are in all biotechnology laboratories. Spinning at enormously high rates separates constituents in a fluid according to density. During leukapheresis, centrifugation is performed to obtain a kind of layering of different white blood cells. The layer taken is that which has a high content of dendritic cells. Dendritic cells are great antigen presenting cells, as Steinman showed us.

The next step is the critical step, and that is to present the dendritic cells with an antigen. The Sip-T process uses a protein from a recombinant fusion-gene (two genes connected together) protein PA2042. The protein has two major pieces. One part is prostatic acid phosphatase (PAP) protein and the other part is granulocyte–macrophage colony stimulating factor (GM-CSF). The GM-CSF protein is a cytokine that is secreted by many immune cells and is used to promote cell growth. The "working" portion is the PAP part. PAP is expressed only in prostate cancer cells or prostate tissue so PAP antigens on PCa cells make them a good target. In fact, PAP was initially used as a biomarker for prostate cancer before the PSA protein was found to be better suited. Its uses as an immunization target goes back to 1997. Initially rats were used to show that vaccination with PAP produced T-cell infiltration of prostate tissue. After rats came men—a step up I hope.

One important point about immunological vaccines is that they do not work quickly; there is a significant lag time. Often with drugs, patients check their PSA frequently after taking the drug, and expect (or hope) to see quick results. It does not work that way with cancer vaccines. It may take six months to obtain a clear noticeable benefit. The immune response however may still be slowing down disease progression. The lag time and reduced rate of progression argue for administering immunotherapy like Sip-T earlier rather than later. Also, if given earlier, the tumor burden is not as great and vaccine have a greater chance to provide a longer lasting, durable response. But early administration is not occurring, as it should. The cost of Sip-T is in the neighborhood of $100,000, so paying for it personally is not possible for most people. Sip-T is FDA approved for asymptomatic or minimally symptomatic mCRPC, so insurance companies likely will cover it only in this progressed stage.

On a negative note, the company that manufactures Sip-T, Dendreon, filed for Chapter 11 bankruptcy in November 2014. Valeant recently purchased the company, so its future looks better. The high cost of the drug, its modest benefit, and the fact that administration of the therapy is cumbersome (compared to a pill or an IV) may have played a role in the original company filing bankruptcy.

Sip-T, Does It Work? Clinical Trials

The primary trial for Sip-T was the Immunotherapy for Prostate Adenocarcinoma Treatment (IMPACT) trial (NCT00065442). It was a double blind study of a total of 512 patients who had metastatic castration resistant prostate cancer. The patients were randomized and either given Sip-T or a placebo. There were twice as many patients in the Sip-T group as the placebo. The regimen included leukapheresis, followed 3-days later by infusion of the activated antigen presenting cells. The regimen is repeated three times, with two weeks in between. The primary end point was overall survival of the patients; that is, how much longer they lived after starting the treatment compared to the placebo group. Patients were enrolled between 2003 and 2007.

The median survival time is the amount of time for 50% of the patients to die. In other words half lived longer and half lived a shorter amount of time. The median survival time of the Sip-T group was 25.8 months vs. 21.7 months for the placebo group. A patient's point of view does not rate this benefit as extraordinary, but a step in the right direction.

206

The main result is that Sip-T did extend survival by 4.1 months.

Another way to view it is to look at the chance of surviving 3 years. For the Sip-T group it is 32% while for the placebo group 23%. Based on the survival increase, the FDA approved Sip-T (Provenge) for mCRPC in 2010, the first immunotherapy approved for any cancer.

A histogram of percent survival in the IMPACT trial at 6 months, 1 year, 2 years, and 3 years is shown in **Figure 13-1.** To a first approximation the Sip-T survival curve is shifted to longer survival times by around 4 months as expected from the median survival times. Notice that the two arms (placebo and Sip-T) give virtually identical survival statistics in the early months. This is a lesson that is being learned over and over again in immunotherapy. There is a lag time for immunotherapy to work. Don't expect immediate improvement. It takes time for your immune system to do its work. Immunotherapy is a tortoise not a hare.

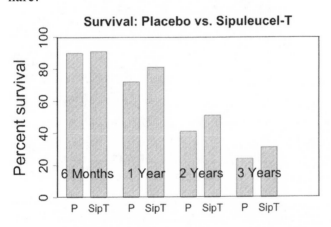

Figure 13-1. Percent Survival curve vs. time on Sipuleucel-T (SipT) or a placebo (P). Notice that at 6 months there is little difference in survival between P and SipT. (Data from PW Kantoff et al., New England Journal of Medicine 365, 411-422 (2010).)

A hazard ratio is often used to quantify results of this type. The simplest version of a hazard ratio is the median survival time of the placebo group divided by the median survival time of the group on therapy, $HR=T_{Placebo}/T_{Sip-T}$. For the IMPACT trial, the hazard ratio was HR = (21.7/25.8) = 0.84. Sometimes people say this results in a 16% reduced risk of death—that is surely a perverse way to state it. The study states a hazard ratio of 0.78 after "adjustments." Hazard ratios are bandied about in the cancer therapy literature and 0.84 or 0.78 are not eye-popping values. Enzalutamide has a hazard ratio of 0.63, and abiraterone 0.75. The flagship vaccine for prostate cancer has some way to go. A patient's perspective is surely different than the researchers'. I'd like to see 0.1 for the HR. Of course, if that is the best we currently have, patients choose to take it. It's like shopping in a former Soviet Union grocery store.

An earlier trial was enacted for patients that were not nearly as advanced as in the IMPACT trial. This was the PROTECT trial (Provenge Treatment and Early Cancer Treatment, NCT00779402) reported in 2011. Its patients were those who were castrate sensitive and recently had a radical prostatectomy for localized prostate cancer. It was a small study with only 176 patients enrolled between 2001 and 2005 with a 2:1 ratio for those receiving Sip-T vs. a placebo. The primary endpoints of this study were the time of biochemical failure and prostate specific antigen doubling time (PSADT). Biochemical failure means when the PSA level of these treated men began to rise and crossed the 3.0ng/ml level.

The results were only moderately encouraging. The time to biochemical failure showed no significant difference between the Sip-T and placebo groups. There was a slight trend for those that experienced biochemical failure that the PSA doubling time was longer in the Sip-T group compared to the placebo group. The important question of whether Sip-T slows down or prevents metastasis was not answered. The median time to metastasis after biochemical failure is 8 years, which is far too long on the scale of this trial. About

16 percent of the patients experience metastasis and of these there was a slight trend suggesting Sip-T patients did better.

Antigen Spreading Observed In Sipuleucel-T

The concept of antigen spreading is a new concept in immunotherapy, and potentially powerful making immunotherapy very attractive. The concept is to target one antigen to kill target tumor cells that then release secondary antigens. The secondary antigens are not specifically targeted by the therapy but they stimulate the immune system to further attack tumor cells. One begins with a narrow attack using one antigen, but the attack broadens to several antigens after their release from the tumor cell. It's like an army that grows in size with every success.

Antigen spreading leads to an adaptable response. As the tumor cells mutate and become resistant to certain therapies, the secondary antigens change as well. But they may also induce a changing immune response. This could be a game changer.

Early signs of antigen spreading appear to have been observed in a report at the American Society of Clinical Oncologists meeting in 2014 in Chicago. The work was led by Charles G. Drake and evaluated the creation of antibodies to secondary antigens for patients treated with Sip-T. The trial was the IMPACT trial (NCT00065442) on patients with metastatic castrate resistant prostate cancer. There were two groups; those receiving Sip-T and a placebo group (2:1). The target antigen was PAP (prostatic acid phosphatase), which is a protein expressed by 95% of prostate cancer cells.

Blood serum was monitored 3-4 months after treatment for antibodies of other cancer antigens. Antibodies in blood serum are a sign your immune system has detected certain antigens. Specifically, immunoglobulin G (IgG) levels of the oncogene K-RAS and of the prostate-specific antigen (KLK2/hK2) were compared between the Sip-T group and the placebo group. The Sip-T group consistently showed elevated antibodies whereas the placebo did not. More importantly, this correlates with increased overall survival. Those Sip-T patients with elevated antibodies greater than twice as large as the placebo group had an overall median survival time of 2.5 times that of those on a placebo.

This is light shining through the thunderclouds. But it does not necessarily prove a clinical benefit, but rather hints at one. However, observations are in line with the theoretical benefits associated with antigen spreading. These ideas open the door to new ways Sip-T and other vaccines can benefit patients. We hope it is a wide door.

Prostvac-VF

Prostvac uses a different means than Sip-T to stimulate the immune system. It uses engineered viruses that contain the DNA with the gene to make PSA protein. This is quite different than Sip-T, which uses your own dendritic cells to carry antigens from the PAP protein. Prostvac, made by Bavarian Nordic, is for use by mCRPC patients.

Viruses are like Trojan horses, releasing their genetic material once inside their victim's cell. Viruses are spherical or tubular bundles of protein and genetic material. They are not alive, yet they infect cells. A virus particle is much smaller than a cell and contains a protein capsid shell (the Trojan horse) in which is stored the genetic material to reproduce the proteins that make up the virus. Viruses use the energy and machinery of the infected cell to reproduce the virus; that is why they are not "alive"—they have no metabolism of their own. The genetic material within the virus capsid can be DNA or RNA depending on the specific virus. The infected cell reads the genetic material carried in by the virus to produce the protein components to make another virus. Philosophers, and us, wonder what the purpose of life is. When considering this question, it may be useful to consider the "life" of a virus. It doesn't even actually live; yet it is programmed to do only one thing and that is reproduce by exploiting others. Seems pointless doesn't it. No joy, no pain, no guts, no glory.

In the Prostvac immunotherapy, the genetic material used in the virus is recombinant. Recombinant means that new genetic material has been added, and these modified genetic materials are called transgenes. The added genetic material does not produce a protein for the virus, but rather will produce protein that contains cancer antigens. The goal is that these antigens are to rattle our immune system. Prostvac uses the PSA protein as the tumor associated antigen. The primary goal is to have the immune system be alerted to this antigen so that it attacks cells that present it; these are of course prostate cancer cells.

The environment around solid tumors often lacks the co-stimulatory molecules to engage the T-cell response. So the Prostvac therapy also includes genes for three co-stimulatory molecules—B7.1, ICAM-1 and LFA-3. The TRIad of COstimualtory Molecules is called TRICOM. We have already encountered the B7 molecule in the context of it being a second signal to activate the T-cell when the APC and T-cell bind. B7 binds to CD28 (CTLA-4). ICAM-1 (CD54) and LFA-3 (CD58) are adhesion proteins that find their way to the surface of the APC. They too bind to the T-cell. The combination of the three co-stimulatory molecules appears to give a response better than just one or any combination of two.

The strategy is a prime plus a boost using two viral agents. Both agents are poxviruses and both are used as vectors meaning they are carriers that bring in the genes to make PSA and TRICOM. The "prime" vaccine is a recombinant Vaccinia virus (Prostvac-V) and the booster virus is a Fowl-pox virus (Prostvac-F); hence the name Prostvac-VF.

What Is The Prime-Boost Strategy?

The vaccinia virus allows large amounts of DNA to be inserted within its capsid. It is a well-studied virus, as it was the vector used in over one billion people for small pox prevention and eradication. The virus itself induces a large anti-vaccinia antibody response. One application of the vaccinia virus, Prostvac-V, produces the primary response. More is better, right? Administering a second dose, however, will be quickly neutralized so that the genes we want expressed will not be expressed. We need something more to expand the response and produce more T-cells that target the PSA antigens. That is the role of the booster virus,

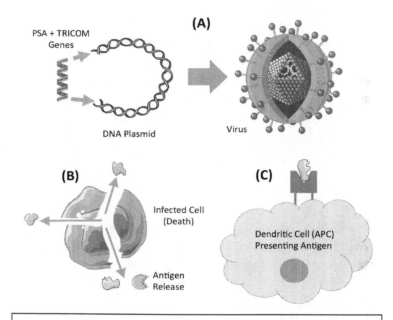

Figure 13-2. The design and action of Prostvac. (**A**) The design of a Prostvac virus. A recombinant DNA molecule containing the genes for PSA+TRICOM genes inserted into a DNA plasmid (circular piece of DNA). This is then inserted into the virus particle. (**B**) The virus infects cells of the patient and upon cell death the infected cell releases antigens of the virus (PSA and TRICOM). (**C**) Antigen presenting cells (APCs) take in the antigens and present them on their surface. This activates T cells to attack cancer cells that express PSA. (More details at CG Drake, Nature Reviews of Immunology 10(8), 580-593 (2010).)

Prostvac-F, which uses a Fowl-pox virus as the vector. Fowl-pox viruses are non-replicating in humans and are not inhibited by antibodies, so repeated doses can be given.

In the Prostvac protocol, the primary dose, Prostvac-V, is given one time, and the booster using Prostvac-F is given six times. All doses have the gene for PSA, the antigen that is targeted for the response.

One might wonder "Why the viruses can cause an immune response to PSA while PSA has been on the cancer cells all along?" Viruses produce a much stronger immune response than that of the cancer cell. The belief is that the vaccinia virus proteins are very immunogenic. They produce an inflammatory environment that enhances the response against this invader, and this includes the PSA protein encoded in the transgene "as a bonus."

Early work using mice showed that the two-virus model enhances the immune response. Work in mice also showed antigen spreading. Mice with tumors that expressed PSA were given Prostvac and the tumors were destroyed. When these mice were reinfected with prostate cancer cells, but this time a strain that did not express PSA, the tumors were also destroyed. Bingo. The interpretation is that destroying the PCa cells releases other antigens that are then targeted by the immune system.

Does It Work In Humans?

There have been eight completed Phase I and Phase II clinical trials with a total of about 300 patients treated. These trials started in 2004, which now is over 10 years ago. They are very time-consuming, considering that patients with mCRPC are in a race against time. Prostvac is well tolerated, and appears that it can be combined with other therapies. Phase 2 trials of combination therapies are underway. General lessons of immunotherapy apply to this vaccine as well—benefit has a time lag, early is better, and low-disease burden is better.

A Phase 2 trial of Prostvac-VF was a blind trial, randomized 2:1. The trial size was small. Eighty-two patients were in the Prostvac-VF arm, and 40 in the control group. The control group received a placebo. Chosen patients had a history of smallpox immunization, had mCRPC with no visceral metastases or severe pain, and no prior chemotherapy. All had a Gleason score of 7 or less. Patients were enrolled between 2003 and 2005.

The primary endpoint was the time of progression free survival (PFS). The mean PFS time was 3.8 months in the Prostvac arm and 3.7 months in the control arm. There was virtually no difference. There were few Prostvac patients who had a PSA response. So far this does not look so positive.

But remember the lag time issues. There was very positive news concerning overall survival. The median survival times were 16.6 months for the placebo arm, and 25.1 months for the Prostvac arm. There was an increase of 8.5 months in survival time. This is very impressive given the lack of progress in treatment for this disease. **Table 13-2** compares the overall survival times of Prostvac-VF with Sip-T immunotherapies. The most meaningful numbers are the increases—comparing the two trials should be done cautiously as the patient populations were not the same.

The Prostvac trial was a Phase 2 trial, and it should be considered preliminary. Its small size may have random biases due to statistical fluctuations in the disease

Table 13-2. Overall survival times (in Months) of two therapeutic PCa vaccines			
	Control arm	Therapy arm	Increase
Prostvac	16.6	25.1	8.5
Sipuleucel-T	21.4	25.9	4.5

progression within the two arms. For example the average age of the two arms of the Prostvac trial were different, 72.6y for the Prostvac arm and 76.8y for the placebo arm. That difference is not insignificant. There were other differences such as PSA values, and levels of hemoglobin, alkaline phosphatase and lactate dehydrogenase, that were

214

more favorable for the Prostvac arm. Likely these differences are not responsible for the large difference of 8.5 months in overall survival between the two groups. Phase 3 trial hopefully will give definitive answers.

A phase 3 trial was initiated in 2011 with the final collection of primary outcome data to be completed by December 2015. The trial is called PROSPECT (NCT01322490) and is led by Drs. Gulley (National Cancer Institute) and Kantoff (Dana-Farber Cancer Institute). It too is for mCRPC patients and it has 1200 patients and is currently ongoing. It has 3 arms; Prostvac-VF + GM-CSF, Prostvac-VF + placebo, placebo + placebo. The 3 arms will each have 1/3 of the patients. We will have to wait for results.

Other PCa Vaccines – DCVAC, DCVax, BPX-201

There are many other groups working on therapeutics PCa vaccines and we mention some of them here.

DCVAC/PCa has similarities with Sip-T in that it modifies the patient's dendritic cells. It has an unusual method for obtaining the antigen. The technique applies high-pressure to PCa cells (in the laboratory) for several hours and this makes them go through apoptosis. This is a nice cross-disciplinary application at a crossroads between biology and physics. Apoptosis is programmed cell death. One of the avoidance tricks cancer cells pull is an avoidance of apoptosis—they do not die-off as they should. Apoptosis is a natural process, and when it occurs cells break up and release all their protein products including antigens. This apoptotic process represents a more natural release of antigens and other molecules. Dendritic cells take up the antigens and present them on their surface to stimulate T-cells.

The pressures used are extremely high, about 150-250 megapascals (MPa). The pressure at the depth of the deepest part of the ocean is about 110MPa. At these high pressures it is found that cells express many of the genes that occur when they go through apoptosis, and then they die. This technique can be used on many types of cancer cells. There is an additional important point—dendritic cells exposed to immunological cell death are exposed to many antigens within the cell, not just one (such as PAP in Sip-T, or PSA as in Prostvac-VF). A single antigen possibly allows for "immune escape," where a specific cancer clone does not express that antigen.

The cells subjected to high pressure are LNCaP cells. These prostate cancer cells are generally used in the laboratory to test drugs and to produce cancer tumors in animals. They are a human prostate cancer cell line that is still androgen sensitive. They were obtained from prostate cancer patients nearly forty years ago, and express PSA.

DCVAC is made by SOTIO located in Prague, Czech Republic. Several Phase 1 and 2 clinical trials have taken place in Europe. A phase 3 trial enrolled its first US patient in late 2014 and its first patient in Europe (Hungary) in May 2014. The trial is called VIABLE (NCT02111577) and will test DCVAC/PCa versus a placebo in mCRPC patients eligible for chemotherapy.

DCVax-Prostate (not to be confused with DCVAC) also modifies a patient's dendritic cells. The antigen used is prostate specific membrane antigen (PSMA). This antigen is also used in engineered gene therapy (Chapter 15), and is a protein expressed in most mCRPC cells. DCVax is a technology used for several cancers, but usually they use cancer cells from the solid tumors of patients to obtain antigens. Metastatic prostate cancer to the bone presents a challenge to obtain a patient's prostate cancer cells. So they use a "generic" antigen such as PSMA. The antigens used in the other vaccines we've discussed also are NOT taken from the patient. Instead it is the dendritic cells that come from the patient. DCVax is manufactured by Northwest Biotherapeutics. Its Phase 3 trial, NCT00043212, has been withdrawn prior to enrollment. This effort appears stumbling.

Another cancer vaccine, GVAX, uses two cell lines, LNCaP and PC3, from which to obtain antigens. The cells have been modified to also express GM-CSF. LNCaP are castrate sensitive, while PC3 are castrate resistant cells. As in other PCa vaccines, the cells are not of the patient. The cells are irradiated causing cell death due to apoptosis. Having two cell lines and using whole cells minimizes the possibility of "immunological escape." A retrospective analysis has found 33 antigens in Phase 1 and 2 trials of GVAX.

The GVAX-PCa concept appears to be a winner, but there have been major stumbles. Phase 1 and 2 trials were positive, but Phase 3 trials reported problems. Two trials, VITAL-1 and VITAL-2, were halted early. The VITAL-2 compared GVAX-PCa + Docetaxel (chemo drug) with Docetaxel alone. Patients were mCRPC, and symptomatic, so they had very advanced disease. Mortalities were not in favor of the combination therapy. A review of the results in August 2008 resulted in an immediate termination of the trial that had started in 2005. This is before dosing levels of Docetaxel were known in combination therapy, and is possibly the cause. Similarly, the VITAL-1 trial, which compared GVAX-PCa alone to Docetaxel alone, was also halted. Suspicions were now aroused which produced increased scrutiny. The trial had started in 2004 and was halted in October 2008 when it appeared likely that it would not meet its overall endpoint of increased survival. This trial was comparing GVAX to a drug that had a known survival benefit. There was no placebo group. It was taking a big leap of faith and daring. We now know much more about PCa immunotherapy and what to expect and not to expect.

Finally, we mention BPX-201, also a dendritic cell vaccine that started a Phase 1 clinical trial (NCT01823978) in 2013. The enrollment includes 18 patients. This new vaccine has a long way to go. Hopefully we will hear more about it in the future. In this vaccine, the dendritic cells are matured, then engineered to express the PSMA antigen and a cell signaling switch. The hypothesis is that the switch is activated at a critical time when the immunotherapy will be most effective. Also given will be an activating agent drug AP1903. Bellicum Pharmaceuticals is the manufacturer.

References

The cancer vaccine roller coaster, B Goldman and L DeFrancesco, Nature Biotechnology 27, 129-39 (2009).

Prostate cancer as a model for tumour immunotherapy, CG Drake, Nature Reviews of Immunology 10(8), 580-593 (2010).

Induction of tissue-specific autoimmune prostatitis with prostatic acid phosphatase
immunization: implications for immunotherapy of prostate cancer, L Fong, CL Ruegg, D Brockstedt, EG Engleman, and R Laus, Journal of Immunology 159, 3113–3117 (1997).

Sipuleucel-T Immunotherapy for Castration-Resistant Prostate Cancer, PW Kantoff, CS Higano, ND Shore, ER Berger, EJ Small, DF Penson, , CH Redfern, AC Ferrari, R Dreicer, RB Sims, Y Xu, MW Frohlich, and PF Schellhammer, and the IMPACT Study Investigators, The New England Journal of Medicine, 365, 411-422 (2010).

Randomized Trial of Autologous Cellular Immunotherapy with Sipuleucel-T in Androgen-Dependent Prostate Cancer, TM Beer, GT Bernstein, JM Corman, LM Glode, SJ Hall, WL Poll, PF Schellhammer, LA Jones, Y Xu, JW Kylstra, and MW Frohlich, Clinical Cancer Research 17, 4558-4567 (2011).

C. Drake, Journal Clinical Oncology 32, Sup 4 Abstract 88 (2014). Presented at the ASCO 2014 Chicago Meeting.

Diversified prime and boost protocols using recombinant vaccinia virus and recombinant non-replicating avian pox virus to enhance T-cell immunity and antitumor responses, JW Hodge, JP McLaughlin, JA Kantor and J Schlom, Vaccine 15, 759-768, (1997).

TRICOM Vector Based Cancer Vaccines, CT Garnett, JW Greiner, K-Y Tsang, C Kudo-Saito, DW Grosenbach, M Chakraborty, JL Gulley, PM Arlen, J Schlom and JW Hodge, Current Pharmaceutical Design 12, 351-361 (2006).

High hydrostatic pressure induces immunogenic cell death in human tumor cells, J Fucikova, I Moserova, I Truxova, I Hermanova, I

Vancurova, S Partlova, A Fialova, L Sojka, P-F Cartron, M Houska, L Rob, J Bartunkova and R Spisek, International Journal of Cancer 135, 1165–1177 (2014).

Elucidating immunologic mechanisms of PROSTVAC cancer immunotherapy, SJ Mandl, RB Rountree, TB dela Cruz, SP Foy, JJ Cote, EJ Gordon, E Trent, A Delcayre and A Franzusoff, Journal for Immunotherapy of Cancer 2:34, 1-13 (2014).

Overall Survival Analysis of a Phase II Randomized Controlled Trial of a Poxviral-Based PSA-Targeted Immunotherapy in Metastatic Castration-Resistant Prostate Cancer, PW Kantoff, TJ Schuetz, BA Blumenstein, LM Glode, DL Bilhartz, M Wyand, K Manson, DL Panicali, R Laus, J Schlom, WL Dahut, PM Arlen, JL Gulley, and WR Godfrey, Journal of Clinical Oncology 28, 1099–1105 (2010).

Prostate cancer vaccines - Update on clinical development, SM Geary and AK Salem, OncoImmunology 2(5), e24523-1, 8 (2013).

Proposed mechanisms of action for prostate cancer vaccines, SM Geary, CD Lemke, DM Lubaroff and AK Salem, Nature Reviews Urology 10, 149-160 (2013).

Chapter 14

Infiltrating the Enemy Whose Name Is Trouble

"You only live once, but if you do it right, once is enough."
Mae West

The following is a most peculiar story. It's a story about what is possible. We get a peek into the future of cancer therapy and it gives us hope. It is not a story of prostate cancer but of bile duct-liver-lung cancer, which involves just one patient. Although these are very limiting aspects, breakthroughs sometimes start quite modestly.

The story involves a mother of six from Billings, Montana (patient 3737) and researchers from the National Cancer Institute. The cancer involved is that of epithelial cells, which are lining cells of membranes. Prostate cancer usually occurs in epithelial cells. Cancer of epithelial cells is what kills most cancer sufferers.

Cancer cells are mutated from normal cells. These mutations cause the cells to ignore instructions and become renegades. Just as important, they refuse to die by normal means. The self-sacrificing apoptosis mechanism of dying to make room for new cells, or to remove themselves when something goes wrong is lost.

Immune cells, lymphocytes including T-cells, infiltrate cancer tumors. What are they doing there? The infiltrating cells are there to attempt to fight the cancer. But they are not winning. Infiltrating cells are checking out these cancer cells and are trying to help the situation. Lymphocytes are not well equipped to attack *self-cells*, which is what cancer cells start out as. But cancer cells are different because of the mutations of the genes of the cell.

But T-cells can and do identify and attack cancerous cells. There is now evidence that T-cells can identify cancer "self" cells by their mutations and consider them "non-self" so they can mount an attack. In May 2014 at the National Cancer Institute, a branch of the National Institutes of Health, scientists carefully studied the infiltrating cells of a tumor (called TIL, tumor infiltrating lymphocytes) and found that they indeed recognize the mutation(s) of a cancer tumor. Steven A. Rosenberg led the work; he is a true giant in cancer research. Dr. Rosenberg had been working on TIL since the 1980s.

The news is exciting, but their technique has been applied to only one patient. The patient had a gastrointestinal cancer that metastasized to the lung and liver. The treatment is ongoing, but so far, the results are very encouraging. The tumors of the patient have been shrinking and have done so for over six months. One cannot predict the future, but without this treatment the future was very dim.

The essence of the treatment is to infuse the patient with very specific T-cells, T-cell that specifically recognize the mutant cancer cells. The mutation only occurred in cancer cells and does not exist in other cells of the patient's body so is a perfect target for these very specific attacking T-cells. To find the very specific T-cells, the genome of the cancer cells had to be sequenced. By comparing with a "normal" genome, mutations of the cancer cells are identified. Once this is known, T-cells of the patient were grown in large numbers outside the body. Infusing these back into the patient in massive numbers produced the desired effect—killing of the cancerous tumor cells. In essence, the patient was given a large dosage of T-cell that initially was infiltrating the tumor and is known to attack the tumor. But now the number of T-cells is so high that the attack is more successful. The process will become clear as we move along.

Let's look at the protocol for this treatment. The protocol will not initially make sense until it is full explained. It is listed up-front so that you will get a sense of where we are going, and that it is not too difficult. (All things seem not so difficult when pioneers blaze the trail for you.)

Here is the protocol for this therapy:
1. Take out some tumor cells and seek mutations that have occurred in these cells that make them different from normal cells.
2. Produce a piece of RNA that combines all the mutations into one sequence. Actually divide the problem up into thirds—divide and conquer. Make three RNA molecules that have the information to generate all the protein fragments that have the mutations.
3. Transfect antigen presenting dendritic cells with the mutation containing RNA.
4. Remove from patient some tumor infiltrating lymphocytes
5. By divide and conquer, determine which mutation(s) of the cancer cell are producing a response in the T-cells.

We are not yet finished, but where are we at so far? We know the mutations that exist in the cancer cell, we have made cells present antigens of the mutations on their surface, and we have determined what the patient's TILs are responsive to. The next phase is to use this information to attack the patient's tumors. If we can determine what the T-cells are responding to in the cancer, we can use this to help destroy the cancer.

Protocol continued:
6. Grow the TILs from the patient in the laboratory, about 10 billion of them along with other T-cells.
7. Inject them into the patient and monitor the response over many months.
8. When tumors are re-occurring (in patient 3737, repeat step 6 but increase the dose twelve-fold to 120 billion T cells.
9. The experiment continues, with regression continuing for a couple of months as the results are reported.

To understand this protocol, we must recall the role of proteins and the central dogma of biology. DNA within each cell contains the code of life, but that information has to be passed on and processed to make proteins. Proteins are the machines of the body. They are made by cells and form the machines; transporters, enzymes, structural and defensive.

Although mutations occur in the DNA, these mutations lead to changes in proteins causing them not to fold into their proper shape and/or to function properly. Structure and function are intimately tied. The central dogma of biology is that DNA is transcribed into RNA, and RNA is translated into protein. Enzymatic protein machines do the work of these seemingly impossible transcription and translation tasks. The key point here is that a change in the DNA code (that is a mutation) produces a change in the RNA, which then produces a change in the protein. Many times these changes are harmless, but in others they are deadly.

What has occurred in this experiment? A patient, named 3737, was infused with T-cells that infiltrated her tumors. The T-cells that were infused were very specific T-cells. They responded to one of the mutations of her cancer cells. The first round of treatment produced an (almost) immediate drop in her cancer burden. This lasted for approximately 6-12 months. Then her tumors began growing again, at least some of her tumors specifically in her lungs. A second treatment, 18 months after the first treatment, was applied. This time with a 12-fold increased dose of T-cells— this resulted in a tumor burden dropping instantly. The tumor burden is still dropping at this time, a few months after the second treatment.

The treatment has been going on for two years, and in the cancer world, this is a huge advance. Drug companies try to shake the world when four months of benefit occurs. The treatment is experimental, and involves an n of 1. Nevertheless, this may show us the way forward.

Its high-tech biotechnology, and although it seems difficult, the procedure is not that difficult (once the trail is blazed). However, it is time consuming and personal for each patient. The difficulty is determining how to use the tools of biotechnology to produce life changing events.

Let's now examine some of the steps in the protocol

more fully so we understand the science involved. It's not that you are to become a biotechnologist that will perform these steps; this set of steps is new, and they will change. If we can understand the steps as they currently are, we can appreciate and understand the further changes and advances that will come. I feel confident in that.

1. Take out tumor cells and determine the mutations.

This step is the foundation of individualized medicine. Individualized medicine is the hope of future patient care, and this is an example of its humble arrival. The idea here is to sequence the DNA of the individual and identify mutations, which sometimes are simply a single letter in the genetic code. The genetic code has just 4 molecular letters: A, T, G, and C. These four molecules are arranged in a long string, and two strings are intertwined into the double helix of DNA. Chapter 6 gives a more complete description of DNA, genes and proteins.

It all starts by reading the DNA in the genome. We have databases of what it is supposed to look like, so it is read to find variations, which are mutations. For patient 3737, there were 26 mutations found. Some of these may be harmful, some not. These mutations are different than normal healthy cells. This makes certain proteins seem foreign, but not too foreign. The great preponderance of the DNA chain is fine and just a few proteins are affected. Maybe they change the protein in a disastrous way to produce cancer, or maybe they change nothing.

The sequencing was done using "whole-exome-sequencing." An exon is that portion of DNA that contains a gene. The collection of these is the exome. The exome is only a small portion of the entire DNA strand. So a whole exome sequence determines the sequence of the entire gene-coding part of the DNA. The cells that were sequenced were taken from the lung. Later we will see that using these cells ultimately led to a treatment that also worked well on the patient's liver tumors. In fact, liver tumor cells were responding better to the treatment than the lung cells that formed the basis of the treatment.

2. RNA of the mutations is made.

The mutation regions were binned into three groups. Each group had roughly a third of the mutations. There were small fragments of the genes fused together to make one large artificial RNA sequence called a tandem minigene. The idea here is to test whether any of these fragments, when they are translated into protein fragments, are seen as "foreign" and elicit an immune response from the patients infiltrating T-cells.

3. Transfect dendritic cells with the RNA.

Dendritic cells are amazing. They gobble up foreign proteins and cut them up into bits. They present them on their surface so that T cells can see their treasure. If the T-cell receptor is able to identify it, it will elicit an immune response. To have all this occur, we must get the RNA into the dendritic cell so that it can produce the mutated protein. Inserting the RNA is done through a process of transfection. Usually this is done by applying a voltage across the cells that causes them to momentarily form pores on their surface membrane made of lipids. Pores allow highly charged external molecules like RNA to enter. It is a quick process, so that the contents within the cell do not have time to escape. The transfected cell now has this RNA with the mutations in it and goes to work expressing the protein encoded by the RNA (which was originally encoded by the DNA). The transfected dendritic cells now present these foreign protein fragments on their surface on the MHC molecule. It's a normal part of the immune response. The big question is "Are there any T-cells floating around that recognize these fragments of protein?" That is answered by the next step.

4&5. Adding infiltrating T-cells from the patient.

The T cells are exposed to the dendritic cells to test whether or not they elicit a response. A response is checked for in the three fragments separately—a divide and conquer strategy. Fragments 2 and 3 were found to elicit no response. Thus 17 of the 26 proteins have been eliminated as having an immune response from the patient. The first fragment, which has 9 of the mutations, does elicit a response. So we are down to 9 suspects out of the 26. Detective work comes into play now. Nine different fragments are made; each fragment has one of the mutations eliminated. They all elicited a response, except one. The one fragment that did not elicit a response had the mutation for a gene ERBB2IP. Bingo. This is the information being sought. The mutation in the ERBB2IP gene is the gene, and the only gene of the 26 that is eliciting a natural immune response. One is not large a large number, but it is infinitely greater than zero and gives enough to move forward.

What about this one gene? The 805'th amino acid in the protein chain for the erbb2 interacting protein (ERBB2IP) is altered from Glutamic Acid to Glycine. (The mutation is denoted E805G, where E is the symbol for Glutamic Acid and G is the symbol for Glycine. See Chapter 6.) A person's life lies on the line, and it's because one crumby amino acid in spot 805 is wrong!

Let's summarize where we are. There were 26 mutations noted in the cells of the patient. Any, all, or none of them could have elicited an immune response. By allowing the infiltrating T-cells to come in contact with the antigens of these mutations, it was found that only one of the 26 produced a response in the patient's immune system. But the patient's immune system is responding to at least one; one is enough. It is this information that is used to treat the patient.

6. Amplify the number of cells.

We now know which T cells are responding to the cancer cells, and we even know to which antigen they are responding. The next task is to harvest some of these cells from the patient, and grow them in large numbers and insert them back to the patient. It is important to note that the T-cells are not altered—they are coming from the patient. They are being expanded in number to produce a sort of enhanced immune response. This has side effects, and can cause sickness.

7. Inject them into the patient and monitor the response.

The first injection included 10 billion of these T-cells **that recognize the mutation.** There were a little over 40 billion T-cells injected and about 25% are of the type that recognize the mutation as foreign. The patient's cancer regressed considerably. Monitored were tumors in the lung and liver. Both organs reduced their burden by about 30% after 6 months. After that, the liver remained steady and the tumor burden in the liver reduced slowly by about 60% after 1.5 years. Unfortunately after 6 months the lung tumors began increasing. After about one year the tumor burden in the lungs was about the same as before treatment started, and increased 20% more after 1.5 years.

8. Repeat injection with higher dosage of mutation responsive T-cells.

After about a year and a half, the process is repeated with 120 billion T-cells that recognize the mutation. This is 12 times the initial treatment and few other (less than 5% total) of other T-cells were injected. The therapy is becoming more targeted. The tumor burden shrunk immediately in the lungs. After nearly two years, the lung tumor burden is on a downward trend, and is about where it was when the treatment started. The liver tumors have done even better. Instead of remaining at a steady level, they dropped at a slow but steady rate.

9. The "experiment" continues.

As of May 2014, the patient has been on therapy for 2 years. This now puts you in the scientist driver's seat. What would you do next? Of course to answer this question depends on how the patient responds to the second infusion, and how long it takes for the cancer to start progressing again, if it does progress.

Protocols that might come to mind are (i) increase the dose further, (ii) give lower doses in an extended schedule (say 6 months), or (iii) give very low doses frequently (every 2 weeks or monthly).

This "infiltrating the enemy" therapy has advantages. It uses the patient's natural immune response to fight cancer, does not alter cells of the patient, making it sort of a natural therapy. Its disadvantage is that the whole-exome-sequencing has to be performed. Or does it? Although we understand the process now that 26 mutations produced only one mutation that the immune system is responding to. But what if we had just infused large amounts of infiltrating T-cells into the patient without knowing this? The same result may have occurred.

Generalizing to other patients, other mutations, other epithelial cancers like prostate cancer may act differently. Surely the mutations will be different from patient to patient. We do not know if the results of the "infiltrating the enemy" experiment are typical or not. Perhaps infiltrating T-cells generally do not recognize mutations, and the current experiment was just a fortunate coincidence. On the other hand, maybe this experiment was unusual in that only one mutation was recognized. Perhaps a more typical example is that several are recognized which would make the therapy more powerful and potent. Onward and upward; there are miles to go before we sleep.

References

Cancer immunotherapy based on mutation-specific CD4 + T cells in a patient with epithelial Cancer, E Tran, S Turcotte, A Gros, PF Robbins, Y-C Lu, ME Didley, JR Wunderlich, RP Somerville, K Hogan, CS Hindrichs, MR Parkhurst, JC Yang, SA Rosenberg, Science 344, 641-645 (2014).

Chapter 15

Engineering T-Cells to Attack Trouble

Where the telescope ends, the microscope begins. Which of the two has the grander view? Victor Hugo

The appearance of advanced metastatic prostate cancer means that the immune system has failed. The cancer cells have avoided or rendered harmless the immune system to destroy them. But the immune system is too powerful to just give up on. Perhaps your T-cells can be altered and given a second attempt at attacking the tumors. One way to do this is by gene engineering the T-cell. Gene engineering means some additional DNA is added to the DNA of the T-cell to produce new proteins that help T-cells attack the tumor. It does not mean rebuilding all the genes of the T-cell. Instead we add just a few more to make it more effective, like adding features to your new truck to make it off-road ready.

Gene therapy sounds scary and a healthy person will want to pass on any thought of this. But for a dreadful disease like metastatic PCa, it offers hope the same way an engineered heart component evokes hope. But there are miles to go before we sleep. The question is can we get there soon enough?

Standard therapies work on the tumor, so moving to the immune system instead to do the work is a gross change in strategy. The immune system is there to defend against invaders. But there are hurdles to overcome to have them recognize and attack cancer cells. Cancer cells are stealth. They have an effective system to not be noticed. In addition their immediate environment is adjusted and made to enhance their ability to hide from killer cells and enhance their survival.

The idea of engineering genes of T-cells to attack cancer is to alter YOUR T-cells so that they attack YOUR cancer. Your cancer cells have specific antigens on them that a T-cell can recognize. We just have to show T-cells the way. They are our Navy Seals performing a surgical attack on cancer lesions.

A strategy of gene therapy is to fine-tune the hunter T-cells to chase down the tumor cells. The hunter's weapon is the T-cell receptor. In gene therapy this receptor is designed specifically for an antigen on the tumor cell. This finely tuned weapon is a chimeric antigen receptor (CAR). A chimera, from Greek mythology, is a creature made up of a mixture of several species—part lion, part goat, and part snake. The chimeric antigen receptor is made of several parts with the hunting element made of an antibody end, a CD8 protein complex of a cytotoxic T-cell, and additional signaling proteins. We will get into the details soon.

There has been success with gene engineered T-cells with chimeric antigen receptors. It starts with mouse models, but there has also been some success in humans. One example is for leukemia—chronic lymphatic leukemia (CLL) and acute lymphoblastic leukemia (ALL). These cancerous conditions involve B cells, another part of the immune system. Here the chimeric antigen receptor has on its end an antibody-derived protein designed to bind to CD19, which is on the surface of B cells. (CD stands for cluster of differentiation). In a trial of 32 CLL patients, about one half responded to the treatment, and slightly less than one quarter went into complete remission. This is remarkable, for these patients had little hope remaining. It was reported that pounds of tumors were removed.

For ALL patients the results are even more impressive. Of 22 pediatric patients, 86% went into complete remission, and of 15 adult patients, 100% went into complete remission with one patient later relapsing. The trial is fresh, so how long an average remission lasts is not known. In July 2014, the FDA granted breakthrough therapy status to investigational chimeric antigen receptor for relapsed/refractory ALL. Breakthrough status allows further development of the therapy to be expedited. The modified T-cells are referred to as CTL019, a chimeric antigen receptor on T-cells targeting CD19.

The application to prostate cancer is behind the curve. Not only are there miles to go, but also the road is steep. New technologies like this evolve, learning both from the failures and the minor successes. The science moves forward by keeping the successful elements and removing or improving on the failing elements. But as there is so very little going on in this area for PCa, this evolution is going to take time. This is disturbing.

What is the goal of gene-engineered T-cells? The goal is to add genes to your T-cells so that the T-cells produce a T-cell receptor on its surface that is sensitive to an antigen on the surface of a tumor cell. The process is called Adoptive Cell Transfer, and is like adapting the hunter to a specific prey.

Let's get into it slowly. **Figure 15-1** shows a cytotoxic-killer (CD8+) T-cell with a chimeric antigen receptor (CAR) on the surface of T-cell. On the CAR's tip are the "sticky" ends of an antibody labeled scFv (single chain fragment variable). These are designed to adhere to a very specific antigen of our choosing. Of course our choice is an antigen on the surface of a PCa cell. What is obvious, but at the same time shocking, is that there are no middlemen. It is a direct interaction between T-cell and tumor cell. The antigen is not being presented on an MHC molecule as in other T-cell immune events.

It is a direct hunter-prey catch—the T-cell is the hunter and its prey is the tumor cell, or more specifically, an antigen on the surface of the tumor cell that identifies it as a cancer cell.

The T-cell receptor has a part above the T-cell surface, a part within the surface membrane, and a part below the membrane projecting into the T-cell interior. The protein CD3ζ that produces signal 1 will be described below. Don't fret about details yet; for now just note that the receptor is the part that is engineered. The engineering job is to develop the receptor so that it attaches to an antigen of our choice, and we will choose an antigen that is unique, or nearly so, to the tumor cell. We do not actually add the

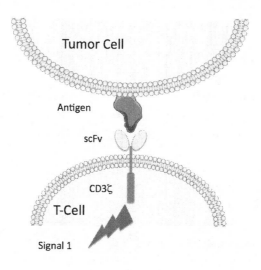

Figure 15-1. An illustration of the binding of an engineered cytotoxic T-cell to the antigen on the surface of a cancer cell. The antigen-binding region of the receptor is designed for a specific antigen and is called the single chain fragment variable (scFv) region, originally from a B-cell. The portions inside the T-cell act to signal the T-cell that it should attack the cancer cell. (More information at MH Kershaw et al., Nature Reviews–Cancer 13, 525-541 (2013).)

receptor to the T-cell—that is far too complicated. All we do is add a section of DNA to the T-cell, and the cell expresses the genes contained within the DNA we add. Expressing the genes means that the protein that makes up the T-cell receptor is manufactured within the cell. Like an instant cake mix, do nothing but add the DNA. It is similar to what a virus does. It adds DNA (or RNA) to a cell to infect it and the infected cell expresses genes to produce more viruses.

Frankenstein it is not. The T-cells are those of the patient. They are first taken from the patient, processed in test tubes, expanded in numbers, and re-infused back into the patient. The key step is that an additional engineered DNA is inserted in the cells. The cells will not be immunologically foreign when reinserted back into the patient since they originally came from the patient. Of course the proteins from the added DNA could be foreign, but that is where careful science must be done.

Frankenstein it is. Unlike drugs or chemotherapy, this therapy is "alive." That presents new challenges. Like Shelly's Frankenstein who turns violent, our engineered T-cells potentially could attack healthy tissue. Only experiments, first with mice then with humans, can prove its safety. The strategy for a trial for liver cancer had to be altered because the T-cell began attacking bile duct epithelial cells. Also, as it is alive, we need to keep it alive. An infusion of engineered T-cells that die off after a week or two may have some use, but we want memory and sustainability in the treatment. Below we will discuss "signal 2" which helps keep the T-cells alive by signaling the T-cells to multiply.

Recombinant DNA

The scary element of the process is the recombinant DNA process. Recombinant DNA is when new genes are inserted within a standard section of DNA to form a new "man-made" piece of DNA. It sounds difficult but in fact is not. The process has been around for a long time. I learned how to do it with bacterial plasmid DNA by recently taking a biotechnology laboratory course at a community college where the average student was 20 years old or so. It's the same process they use to modify corn and other foods to make them resistant to pests or drought.

There are three parts to the process. First is to extract sections of DNA from a source that we wish to insert. One such example is the single-chain antibody variable fragment (scFv) as seen in the previous **Figure 15-1**. This DNA fragment comes from B-cells that express the antibody we wish to use as the sticky-end of the T-cell receptor. DNA fragments can be cut out from a long piece of DNA by using carefully chosen enzymes, called restriction enzymes, and the process is called digestion. There is an industry for these enzymes. Many hundreds are available that cut at specific places and in a specific way. The enzymes usually cut the double helix strand in a way that the two strands are of slightly different lengths, differing by 1-5 bases generally. There is an overhang of one strand relative to the other. This is great if we plan things correctly. We can have a piece we want to attach to it to have a complementary strand. Thus if our first piece has an ATTG overhang, we want the piece to connect to it to have a TAAC overhang. (Remember, A pairs with T, and G pairs with C.) These overhangs are very particular, as DNA does not want to bind to anything but a complementary strand.

The next step is to mend all the pieces together, which is to ligate them. Figure 15.1 shows several proteins (scFv, a linker which includes a hinge and CD8, CD3ζ) strung together. This is achieved by stringing together the DNA sequence for each of these proteins. An enzyme, called a ligase, is used to attach the DNA sequences together. All one does is add the ligase to a mixture at a working temperature for a specific time. The process may be stepwise ligating each portion sequentially. It's the planning that is important, as each digestion-ligation step has to fit together, including a Lego-block-like attaching of DNA strands that have overhangs due to the differing lengths of the two DNA strands during digestion.

It is a lot of work to do this, but once it's done it's done. The final step is to duplicate our work on a kind of DNA copying machine. The DNA copy process is the polymerase chain reaction, or PCR. The process is called amplifying DNA and was the subject of the 1993 Nobel Prize in Chemistry, which went to Kary B. Mullis *"for his invention of the polymerase chain reaction (PCR) method."* Mullis is quite a character and is usually pictured with his surfboard in California. The point is that once one makes a tiny bit of desired DNA sequence, one can make plenty more in just 2-3 hours. A simple machine does most of the work and is programmed to cycle three different temperatures multiple times. The first temperature melts the DNA (separating the two strands of the double helix). Next the temperature is reduced to allow "primer annealing." In solution is a short "primer" strand containing a handful of bases (e.g. AAGTCA), which are designed to attach (anneal) at the end by making it complementary to the existing DNA strand. For example, the primer used to make the light chain variable section of the CAR to bind to prostate PSMA is 5'-AAC ACT CAT TCC TGT TGA AG-3'. DNA is directional, which is indicated by the 3' and 5' ends. The third and final temperature segment in each cycle grows the rest of the strand by adding one base at a time until it reaches the end. The growing is done at high temperature (e.g. 95°C), and is accomplished by an enzyme, DNA polymerase. The whole process occurs inside a small closed test tube. This sequence of events is repeated many times, say 30, and each time the number of strands doubles, at least in theory. The sequence is $1, 2, 4, 8, 16, \ldots\ldots 2^{30}$, so after 30 cycles we have $2^{30} = 1.09$ billion. Of course everything can and will go wrong. But once the technique is mastered for a specific system, lots of product should result.

The lesson here is that once the ideal T-cell receptor is "designed" and once a DNA strand is made, we can make much more of it cheaply and quickly. If such a prefect receptor is made for prostate cancer, it could be used on thousands of patients without much extra effort in this phase of the project.

Of course there is the next issue of getting the DNA into each patients T-cells. This can be done by electroporation (a high voltage drives the highly charged DNA inside) or by using an inert viral package with the desired DNA inside it. Usually a virus package is used. The outer shell of a virus, its viral capsid, is a spherical like protein shell. Within it is genetic material used to infect the cell. The virus package is made harmless by removing the harmful genetic material and instead inserting the desired DNA. Viruses are experts at adding DNA or RNA to cells, so we hijack the infection capability of a virus, and instead infect ourselves with DNA that will cause the cell to express the chimeric antigen receptor.

The Design Of The Receptor

The chimeric receptor has many jobs. The first task is to find a cancer cell with the surface antigen that we have programmed the T-cells to adhere to and bind to it. The ideal is for the antigen to exist only on the cancer cell so that only cancer cells are targets. This is the primary job of the part external to the T-cell, the so-called binding domain of the CAR. It is composed of a piece of an antibody, the so-called single chain variable fragment (scFv, see **Figure 15.1**). Recall that the variable part of an antibody is the portion that is able to identify a specific antigen. B-cells make antibodies and each B-cell makes an antibody where the variable is for one antigen, and only one. Thus we need an scFv that will attach to the cancer cell. The scFv portion of the CAR is like a magnet that sticks to just one thing—the antigen target. Antigen targets for prostate cancer are discussed below.

The receptor runs through the T-cell membrane into the interior where signaling occurs. These signals tell the T-cell that it has made contact with the enemy. This part of the CAR is intracellular and is the signaling domain of the CAR. Signals instruct the T-cell to begin expression of genes that are specific for the task of activating the T-cell to attack.

There are three potential signals. The protein CD3ζ shown in **Figure 15.1** produces the first signal, called signal 1. This is the primary signal and CAR designs with just these elements are call "first generation." Work on these started in the 1980s. The first generation is insufficient to get a full response. In some cases a response will occur but it is short lived before the T-cells become dormant in a state called anergy.

T-cell activation is usually described as occurring from a primary signal and co-stimulatory signaling. The first signal indeed causes the T-cell to become cytotoxic, but we need co-stimulatory signals for the effort to be enduring. A second signal is used to instruct the T-cell to expand its population—that is, to produce more troops to attack the enemy. The third signal is received by cytokine receptors on the surface of T-cells. Cytokines are signaling molecules between cells—a means for cells to communicate. This draws the troops to the battlefield.

Today's research is mainly focused on enhancing signal 2 and signal 3, the co-stimulatory signals after the primary signal. Signal 2 causes a phosphorylation (adding a phosphate group) event to occur after signal 1 is initiated. Phosphorylation is a way to change the function of a protein. Once the initiating signal 2 Phosphorylation event occurs, a cascade of events follows. Phosphorylation is a key signaling strategy in cells where kinase molecules add phosphate groups to molecules. This changes the properties and binding characteristics of the acted on molecule. In the end it leads to expression of genes within the T-cell to grow and attack the tumor. Phosphorylation is a product of the energy molecule adenosine triphosphate (ATP) where a phosphate is removed and deposited elsewhere and ATP becomes adenosine diphosphate (ADP).

The third signal is the release of cytokines. These signaling molecules cause cells to respond in many ways. An important cytokine for T-cells is interleukin 2 (IL-2), a T-cell growth factor. **Figure 15.2** compares normal T-cell activation with 1st and 2nd CAR T-cells.

The challenges, and opportunities, in obtaining productive co-stimulatory signals occur because gene engineered T-cells operate differently than "natural" T-cells. We are trying to play by some new rules. This makes the design difficult since we are not relying on the rules of the natural method. The rules that natural T-cells go by are that they adhere to antigens presented on the surface of antigen presenting cells (APCs), and the antigen is not there by itself.

Figure 15-2. A comparison of normal T-cell activation with that of T-cell attack of cancer cells using chimeric antigen receptors, CARS. **(A)** The natural activation of T-cells by binding of the T-cell receptor to an antigen presented on the MHC of an antigen presenting cell (APC). The activated T-cell has to then reproduce and hunt for the tumor cell. **(B)** A first generation CAR that by itself is capable of producing Signal 1. Signal 2 requires binding to an APC. **(C)** A 2nd generation CAR that has co-stimulatory proteins in the CAR that alone presents both Signal 1 and Signal 2. Adding proteins to the CAR creates 3rd generations that produce Signal 3 as well. **(B&C)** Note that the tumor cell is directly involved in engineered CAR T-cells, in contrast to the natural process (A). (More details at D W Lee et al., Clinical Cancer Research 18, 2780-2790 (2012).

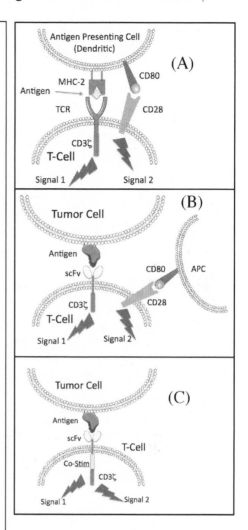

The antigen is processed and presented on the surface by the major histocompatibility complex (MHC) after the cell has processed "foreign" antigens. Here is a big difference; the natural attachment causes other attachments to occur. A form of synapse is formed with CDs on the T-cell surface with other CD molecules on the antigen-presenting cell. This synapse produces the co-stimulatory signal 2 for "free."

Gene engineered T-cells do not rely on the MHC but bind directly with the antigen, which results in a loss of signal 2. A solution of this problem was discovered in 1998. The solution was to fuse genes together so that those of the T-cell receptor are in tandem with those of co-stimulatory molecules that form the synapse. Specifically in 1998 the7 gene of CD28 was added to the genes for scFv + spacer + CD3ζ. CD28 is one of the molecules that gets stimulated in the synapse during natural T-cell activation. In the synapse a protein called B7 that is on the antigen-presenting cell activates it.

Fusing these genes simply means that the DNA sequence CD28 is ligated to the DNA sequence of the other genes as discussed in the recombinant DNA section above. There is just one larger gene that is inserted into the T-cell to produce a second generation CAR. The experiments were done in test tubes and the cells were electroporated. It's only a proof of concept. But when an antigen was presented the T-cells responded producing both signal 2 and signal 3. Signal 3 was a 20-fold increase of IL-2 produced by the T-cells. The concept is proven, and variations of this theme are the paradigm for today's experiments in test tubes, mice and humans.

Gene engineered T-cells bind directly to the antigen, which has advantages. One of the ways that cancer cells can avoid destruction by natural T-cells is to down-regulate the production of MHC. If there are no MHC molecules on the surface, antigens are not present on the surface so that natural T-cells never bind to them and no signals, primary or co-stimulatory, are produced. Engineered T-cells do not need MHC and its version of antigen presentation. They bind directly to surface antigens. Only about 20% of antigens are on the surface, but with "smarts" we can find one to do the trick.

Application to Prostate Cancer

Hopefully you have made it this far and are now ready to see how all this applies to prostate cancer in humans, not theoretically in test tubes. Here is a checklist of items that must be identified or results/actions that must occur:

1. The target—An antigen specific to the tumor cell.
2. The weapon—A T-cell receptor that is sensitive to the antigen of the disease. This is a key feature and is where gene engineering comes into play.
3. Loading the weapon—Activation of the T-cell by the antigen.
4. A supply of troops—Maintaining a population of T-cells that will continue the fight.
5. Not getting stuck in mud and mire—Overcoming environmental and epigenetic factors inhibiting the T-cells.
6. Proper tactics -- Outsmarting Immuno-suppressants of diseased cells.
7. No collateral damage—Attack only the diseased cells and not healthy cells.

All items on the checklist must be met to win the war.

The first item is a target, an antigen. For prostate cancer we are lucky. There are several, with three of them being the prostate specific membrane antigen (PSMA), prostate stem cell antigen (PSCA), and TCRy alternate reading frame protein (TARP). Most of the work has used the PSMA antigen. PSMA is a protein (antigen) of 750 amino acids that resides on the surface membrane of prostate cancer cells. PSMA is up regulated by a factor of ten in prostate cancer and is up-regulated further under androgen depravation therapy. Prostate antigens are not foreign, but we want to treat them as such. A radical prostatectomy removes the prostate, so ideally these patients should not have any prostate antigens, although they do due to metastases. However these are all enemies and it's safe to declare them foreign by smart engineering of weaponry.

Note that PSMA is different from PSA, the antigen we are most familiar with to monitor tumor activity. PSA is not used presumably because it circulates in the blood and will "clog" up engineered T-cells far before they ever arrive at a tumor.

The first use of PSMA as a target goes back to 1999. The research was very cautious as it needed to establish some basics that we now take for granted. T-cells were engineered to have a receptor sensitive to PSMA and a CD3ζ fusion receptor. It was far too early to infuse the engineered T-cells into patients. Working in a test tube, good news was found all around—the T-cells attacked (lysed) the cancerous prostate cells. This work showed something fundamental that we now take for granted—and that is the T-cells of PCa patients are up to the job. In science, one must be cautious to assume anything. Five patients with different stages of PCa contributed T-cells, and all of them, when engineered, were competent to bind to PSMA and attack and destroy prostate cancer cells. The stage is set for further advances.

First Generation Experiments

The group that has been chipping away at this steadily is that of Dr. Richard P. Junghans, currently at Roger Williams Medical Center in Providence, Rhode Island. Their work on prostate cancer started in 2004. Just four years earlier new antibodies were developed that bind to the part of PSMA that sticks out from the membrane of a cancer cell, and these were used to make the scFv sticky portion of an engineered T-cell receptor. The design had a hinge (CD8) and CD3ζ. This is a "standard" generation 1 design. T-cells were transfected with the engineered DNA by using a retrovirus. The experiments were performed in test tubes.

T-cells can be monitored for activation by measuring if cytokines (IL-2) are secreted and if the T-cells express CD25. Indeed, both IL-2 and CD25 increase their levels of secretion/expression. This is an early indication that the process works, at least to some level.

This next led to animal tests in mice that were

inoculated with tumor cells. The mice were "nude" mice, which have an inhibited immune system. This allows cancer cells to more aggressively invade. Two types of tumor cells were used: those that expressed PSMA (PSMA+) and those that did not (PSMA-). At the same time they were inoculated with tumor cells, the mice were administered gene engineered T-cells. The mice were monitored for 15 days. Those mice with PSMA- cancer cells grew tumors of about ¼ inch. There was no difference between animals that were administered CARs and those that were not. The engineered T-cells have no effect on PCa if the cancer cells do not express PSMA—no PSMA, no attack by the T-cells.

The results were very encouraging for the PSMA+ mice. Most of the mice in this group (56%) did not grow tumors when also administered the engineered T-cells. And of those that did grow tumors, the growth was either delayed or the rate of tumor growth was far reduced. To add additional credibility that the very positive effect is indeed the result of engineering T-cells, both PSMA+ and PSMA- mice were administered normal (non-engineered) T-cells. These mice grew ¼ inch tumors—convincing evidence that gene engineering is the factor reducing tumors.

At the time of these experiments in 2004, others were on similar trails for brain, liver, melanoma, breast, colon and lung cancers. Each of these has to be treated differently. Obviously the CAR has to have a specific antibody section, the scFv that is dependent on what that cancer cell *uniquely* expresses on its surface. The 2004 experiments of the Junghans group are indeed encouraging and were the first on prostate cancer. They opened the door for treatment in humans and led to clinical trials on a very small number of patients. The results are described below.

Second generation experiments.

The initial experiments on PCa were first generation experiments. This takes us all the way to 2014, when very similar experiments to the 2004 experiments were performed, but using 2nd generation CARs. A co-stimulatory protein CD28 is fused into the gene. This is the same gene fused in much earlier 1998 exploratory work by Finney and coworkers who showed primary and co-stimulatory responses from a fused gene. The results were very encouraging. Three measures were evaluated—the secretion of cytokines, the ability to proliferate T-cells and attack tumor cells that express PSMA, and the effect of tumor cells in mice.

An important consideration is getting the DNA for the CAR within the T-cell—permanently. Fortunately here we can take a lemon and make lemonade. The lemon is the virus, but the lemonade is that the virus can fuse its DNA with your DNA in the T-cell, permanently. A virus in its simplest term is a shell of protein with DNA (or RNA) inside its protective shell. The DNA contains genes that code for the proteins that make it up. There are not that many genes (usually), let's say a dozen different genes. But each gene may need to make many identical copies of the expressed protein to reproduce itself (often a multiple of 60 to make its icosahedral shell of identical proteins). After infecting a cell, the DNA is expressed using the machinery of the infected cell to produce the proteins that usually self-assemble to form more viruses. You heard about all this earlier in different contexts. New here is the concept of a retrovirus. Retroviruses work by infecting a cell and placing the virus DNA not just anywhere, but fusing it with the DNA of the host. Once it is inserted, it is permanently part of the DNA of the T-cell. That's what makes retroviruses, like HIV, so difficult to deal with. But this is our lemonade. When the cell reproduces, it reproduces its entire DNA including the inserted part. The game here is to repackage a harmless retrovirus with the DNA we want expressed, and infect our T-cells with the retrovirus. Very sweet tasting lemonade.

T-cells release cytokines when they bind to the prostate cancer cell. Cytokines are small proteins that are used for signaling. Signaling here means alerting all the other nearby T-cells that they have found their prey, and instructs them to gear up for an attack and increases their propensity to expand their numbers. The two cytokines relevant for this case are IL-2 and interferon gamma (IFN-γ). The 2nd generation CAR was far superior in the secretion of IL-2 and IFN-γ, with a 10-fold increase in secretion compared to the 1st generation CAR.

T-cells, when activated, will be signaled to proliferate; that is to reproduce more T-cells to aid in the attack. These experiments compared the proliferation of groups of T-cells: normal T-cells, generation 1, and generation 2 T-cells. Cells were placed in contact with PSMA+ prostate cancer cells for 3 days and allowed to proliferate for 6 more days (9 days total). Starting with 200,000 T-cells in each group, after 9 days their numbers increased to 520,000 (normal T-cells), 1,640,000 (Generation 1) and 2,580,000 (Generation 2). Note that there was some growth even for normal T-cells (factor of 2.6 increase), but it is meager in comparison to the increases of generation 1 (factor of 8.2) or generation 2 (factor of 12.9). The 2nd generation proliferated most effectively and more quickly.

The most important questions concern toxicity of the T-cells on PSMA+ cancer cells. This was measured in a test tube, and then on mice. The test tube results showed that the 2nd generation T-cells were cytotoxic (cell toxic), but in fact had a toxicity of only 71% that of the 1st generation T-cells. Disappointing it is not—the important point is that the 2nd generation T-cells have not inadvertently become impotent.

More importantly are the results on mice that have been subcutaneously inoculated with PCMA+ prostate cancer cells. This causes tumors to grow in the inoculated mice and are visible to the naked eye in a couple of weeks or less. Two sets of mice were used; one set of mice was irradiated with gamma radiation similar to X-rays, and one set of mice was un-irradiated. The radiation intensity is below lethal doses.

Why radiation? Radiation is a tool to produce lymphodepletion, a reduction of the number of lymphocytes, including T-cells, within the mice. This sounds a bit crazy to knock down the lymphocyte count if one is trying to attack tumor cells. But the immune system is complex—it must be very diverse, yet at the same time it can only handle so many T-cells at once. When the immune system expands during an infection, it sacrifices some of its members in a form of attrition. It is as if room needs to be made for the expanding population of T-cells that are directly involved in the fight. The process is referred to as non-myeloablative conditioning which refers to the absence of severely affecting bone marrow cells to knock down the immune system. This trick seems to work and is a method to make adoptive T-cell transfer more effective. It has been used not only in mice but in human patients as well. Patients receive chemotherapy instead of radiation. Conditioning can change the length of time of survival. That's a big deal.

The results of these experiments on mice were outstanding. First we discuss the irradiated mice, which were lymphodepleted. There were three groups with eight mice in each group. One group was treated with natural T-cells, the second group was treated with the 1st generation CAR, and the final set was treated with the 2nd generation CAR. Mice treated with the 2nd generation CAR did far better than either of the other two groups. The tumor volume of 2nd gen CAR T-cell treated mice was about $1/10^{th}$ that of those administered 1st gen CAR T-cells. Obviously this shows that the 2nd gen CAR T-cells are more robust in their proliferation and attack on tumor cells. To put the results in more stark terms, only 1 of the 8 mice treated with 1st gen CARs showed no signs of tumor growth, while 6 of the 8 2nd gen treated mice showed a complete response. This contrasts with no mice showing no tumor growth when administered normal T-cells.

Similar results were obtained for the non-irradiated mice; with the 2nd generation CAR treated mice responding far better than the 1st gen or the normal T-cell treated groups.

These results are very exciting in that the failure of the immune system to protect against the growth of tumors in mice can be reversed in most cases. But it is difficult to extrapolate these results to humans. First off, response times that lasts two or three weeks is not long enough to know if this is lasting. Secondly, there may have been other very negative effects on the mice that we cannot know about. Finally, we are far larger and more complex than mice to know if there are any positive effects for humans. The only way to know any of this is through clinical trials.

Clinical Trial

A clinical trial was funded in 2005 to use the first generation CAR on advanced prostate cancer. Recall that the 2nd generation T-cells were not developed until 2014, so the trial CARs did not have signal 2 capabilities. Phase I trials are on a small group of patients to determine safety, dosage and side effects. Of course it will also determine if tumors are reduced in size. Recruitment of patients was started in 2007. Funding to Dr. Junghans for the trial was from the U.S. Department of Defense Prostate Cancer Program (PCRP).

This is the first test of a gene-modified T-cell therapy on humans with prostate cancer, so it is important. This trial used lymphodepletion to better the chances that the CAR T-cells will respond properly. This non-myeloablative conditioning was of course not by gamma radiation as in mice, but by a form of chemotherapy. In addition, patients received cytokine IL-2 at low or intermediate doses. Various doses of T-cells were considered -- 1 billion, 10 billion or 100 billion (10^9, 10^{10} or 10^{11} CAR T-cells.).

Expectations were that the CAR T-cell therapy would be well tolerated, that T-cells would attack cancer cells, and that the lymphodepletion will aid in its effectiveness. The big objective is to ultimately "develop a cure for metastatic prostate cancer" and to kill prostate cancer cells anywhere in the body. The trial itself is entitled "Trial of Anti-PSMA Designer T-cells in Advanced Prostate Cancer after Non-Myeloablative Conditioning," NCT00664196/NCT01929239. Anti-PSMA is the term for the antibody (the scFv) that attaches to PSMA.

It is still ongoing and is scheduled to end Dec. 2015.

But there are some preliminary results.

In 2010, there were 4 patients treated. Three were treated at the lowest dose of 10^9 CAR T-cells and one at 10^{10} T-cells. In addition patients were infused with IL-2 at either low dose or high dose. Two of the patients that received the lower CAR dose had significant PSA reductions of 50% and 70% two months following treatment. Unfortunately two of the patients, including one at the high T-cell dosage, had minimal PSA response (less than 20%). Those that did not respond had body IL-2 levels 10-15 times lower than those responding. Thus IL-2 levels are an important part of the therapy. The results are mixed. Fortunately there were no severe side effects from the CAR T-cell therapy itself. There were side effects from the lymphodepletion—fever and neutropenia (low white blood cell count).

The trial took a turn in 2012/2013 and was redesigned to test the role of cytokine IL-2 levels in the treatment. By this time a 5th patient was treated and at the higher 10^{10} CAR T-cell dose. That patient had a minimal PSA response. Science is always full of surprises and the surprise here is that response appears to be correlated inversely with CAR T-cell dose—in other words, higher CAR T-cell infusions yielded poorer outcomes. Positive outcomes correlated with IL-2 levels in blood plasma. Apparently IL-2 levels go up, with better tumor control, with lower levels of CAR T-cell dose. It first seems paradoxical, but the new study design hypothesizes that the higher number of CAR T-cells are absorbing IL-2 (presumably through IL-2 receptors on their surface) and reducing the IL-2 levels below an activation threshold to kill tumor cells. The redesign is to evaluate both the IL-2 dose (low, medium, and high) in conjunction with the dose of CAR T-cells. The goal is to eventually give high doses of 10^{11} CAR T-cells, but currently it is unknown what level of IL-2 is needed to maximize the number of CAR T-cells that are actively attacking tumors. It's a thorny question and takes time to answer but worth it. The goal is a cure.

References

Gene-Engineered T-cells for cancer therapy, Michael H Kershaw, J. A. Westwood and P. K. Darcy, Nature Reviews – Cancer 13, 525-541, (2013).

The Future Is Now: Chimeric Antigen Receptors as New Targeted Therapies for Cancer
DW Lee, DM Barrett, C Mackall, R Orentas, and SA Grupp, Clinical Cancer Research 18, 2780-2790 (2012).

Chimeric Receptors Providing Both Primary and Costimulatory Signaling in T-cells from a Single Gene Product, HM Finney, ADG Lawson, CR Bebbington and ANC Weir, Journal of Immunology 161, 2791-2797 (1998).

Cancer Patient T-cells Genetically Targeted to Prostate-Specific Membrane Antigen Specifically Lyse Prostate Cancer Cells and Release Cytokines in Response to Prostate-Specific Membrane Antigen, MC Gong, J-B Latouche, A Krause, WDW Heston, NH Bander and M Sadelain, Neoplasia 1(2), 123–127 (1999).

Anti-Prostate Specific Membrane Antigen Designer T-cells for Prostate Cancer Therapy, Q Ma, M Safar, E Holmes, Y Wang, AL Boynton and RP Junghans, The Prostate 61, 12-25 (2004).

The homodimer of prostate-Anti-PSMA Designer T-Cells specific membrane antigen is a functional target for cancer therapy, N Schulke, OA Varlamova, GP Donovan, D Ma, JP Gardner, DM Morrissey, RR Arrigale, C Zhan, AJ Chodera, KG Surowitz, PJ Maddon, WD Heston, WC Olson, Proceeding of the National Academy of Science USA 100, 12590–12595 (2003).

Advanced Generation Anti-Prostate Specific Membrane Antigen Designer T-cells for Prostate Cancer Immunotherapy, Q Ma, EM Gomes, A S-Y Lo, and RP Junghans, The Prostate 74, 286-296 (2014).

Phase I trial of anti-PSMA designer T-cells in advanced prostate cancer, RP Junghans, R Rathore, Q Ma, R Davies, A Bais, E Gomes, E Beaudoin, H Boss, P Davol and S Cohen,
Journal of Clinical Oncology, 2010 ASCO Annual Meeting Abstracts, Vol 28, No 15 suppl (May 20 Supplement), 2010: e13614.

Treatment of Metastatic Renal Cell Carcinoma With Autologous T-Lymphocytes Genetically Retargeted Against Carbonic Anhydrase IX: First Clinical Experience
HJ Lamers, S Sleijfer, AG Volto, WHJ Kruit, M Kliffen, R Debets, Jw Gratama, and G. Stoter, Journal of Clinical Oncology, 24, e20-e22 (2006), editorial.

Phase IB trial redesign to test role of IL2 with anti-PSMA designer T-cells to yield responses in advanced prostate cancer, RP Junghans, Journal of Clinical Oncology 30, 2012 (suppl 5; abstr 70, American Society of Clinical Oncology annual meeting).

Role for IL2 adjunctive cotherapy for suppression of a solid tumor with designer T-cells: Phase I trial data in prostate cancer, RP Junghans, Journal of Clinical Oncology 31, 2013 (suppl 6; abstr 216, American Society of Clinical Oncology annual meeting).

Designer immune cells fight prostate cancer: 'Living drug' shows promise in early clinical trials, News, Nature April (2009). doi:10.1038/news.2009.376.

Chapter 16

Einstein Goes After Trouble

This radiation has an analogy in acoustics in the form of the so-called shock waves produced by a projectile or an aeroplane travelling at an ultra-sonic velocity (Mach waves, Sonic Booms). A surface analogy is the generally known bow wave. Pavel Cherenkov, Nobel Prize Lecture 1958.

Nanomedicine is a 21st Century technology being developed to treat cancer. It's so new that it has more promise than it has homeruns. An often-used strategy is to use a nanoparticle as a small vesicle to carry a toxin to an offending cell—a nanoparticle version of the Trojan horse trick. A variation of this theme is photodynamic therapy (PDT), meaning that the nanoparticles are activated by light. Activation by light gives an extra degree of control of what is poisoned. But PDT is of no use if we are trying to act on tumors, such as metastatic prostate cancer, that are deep within the body where light does not penetrate. Add to that the significant complication that often we do not even know where cancer cells are hiding out. So where do we shine the light even if it could get in?

Here is where Professor Einstein shakes hands with nanotechnology, chemistry and medicine. Einstein supplies the physics for cancerous cells to emit light—this produces a cascade of engineered events to kill the cancerous cells. The engineering involves having cancerous cells absorb a molecule with a radioactive atom used routinely as an imaging reagent in PET scans. But as an Einsteinian byproduct, the spewing out of very fast moving particles from the radioactive process produces visible light—light that will not escape your body but simply lights up your cancer cells like a spelunker with a flashlight inside a bat cave. From there we can use our imagination. One imaginative concept is actually simple: use the light to strike nanoparticles that have driven themselves to lodge within cancer cells, which then causes the nanoparticles to create cytotoxins which produce apoptosis or necrosis (death) of the cancer cells. Without light nothing happens. We have some control over when toxicity occurs and which cells receive it.

Let's look at the peculiar way that visible light is produced during a radioactive event. Radioactivity does not produce visible light. Radioactive events often produce (gamma) γ-rays which are a very high energy light ray that one cannot see and that goes right through tissue. This light is not anywhere near visible light and is not of interest for this application. Besides γ-rays, radioactive events also spit out fast moving particles like electrons or its antiparticle positrons. The process is called (beta) β-emission. These particles have mass. Einstein's special theory of relativity produces a backdoor method for very high velocity charged matter to produce visible light. The special theory of relativity, published by Einstein in his wonder year of 1905, connects matter with light and space with time. The matter-light relationship is known by all, $E=mc^2$, where m is the mass of the matter and c is the speed of light. This relationship gives the amount of energy contained in mass. A 1 kg (2.2lb) mass, if converted entirely into energy is about 10^{17} Joules of energy. This is enough to power a 655MW electrical power plant for about 5 years. This famous relationship is for a stationary mass. The energy of a mass moving at speed v is $E = mc^2/(1-v^2/c^2)^{1/2}$. The energy of the moving mass includes both its rest energy and its kinetic energy. A mass moving at 0.99c has energy of $7mc^2$. More importantly, as v approaches c the energy becomes infinite. It takes an infinite amount of energy for a massive object to travel at the speed of light. For particles with mass, it is impossible to travel at c or above.

Radioactive nuclei emit particles that travel at very high speeds, sometimes approaching c but always less than c. But this is where the first weirdness sets in. In a material medium, light slows down and travels at a speed less then c. Glass and water are examples of media in which light slows down. In glass, light travels at about 2/3 c, and in water it travels at about ¾ c. This change of speed causes light to bend giving the image that a stick inserted into a swimming pool appears broken, and in glass this bending of light is used to form lenses. This first weirdness is not so weird after all.

We have an interesting situation here, producing the second weirdness. Particles from radioactive decay cannot go faster than light, but they can go faster than light in a medium such as glass or water—or in the medium of interest, tissue of the human body. To see what happens in this case, one has to go further with special relativity and use the four laws of the electricity and magnetism known as Maxwell's equations (first discovered during the American Civil War in 1865). One finds that a particle traveling faster than the local speed of light emits electromagnetic radiation (light) to slow it down. The radiation is called Cherenkov radiation after its discoverer, Pavel Cherenkov (also spelled as Cerenkov). The discovery was made in 1934 and he received the Physics Nobel Prize in 1958. It is the source of a beautiful blue colored glow of water in tanks surrounding nuclear reactors. Therefore, matter can travel faster than light if the light has been slowed down by a medium. Then the matter, if electrically charged, produces a "glow."

Scientists at Washington University in St. Louis in early 2015 have developed a technique to use visible/UV Cherenkov radiation in a form of photodynamic therapy for cancer. They used their imagination combining nanomedicine with light produced in your body from a radioactive source. It is this combination that we describe here. This is a futuristic method. It has so far only been tested in a Petri dish and on mice. The major players in the development are shown in **Table I**.

Table I. The players	
β^+ (Positron) β^- (Electron)	Beta particles. The positron is the antiparticle of an electron. These high-speed particles emit UV-visible Cherenkov light.
TiO_2 (Titanium dioxide)	A solid crystalline material with light-responsive chemical catalytic properties.
$nTiO_2$ (nano titanium dioxide)	A nanoparticle of TiO_2, say 18nm in diameter.
FDG (^{18}F)fluoro-deoxyglucose	A molecule very similar to glucose but with a radioactive Fluorine attached that emits positrons that produce Cherenkov light. Cells with high metabolism, like cancer cells, take up FDG. Commonly used in PET scans.
Tf (Transferin)	A protein that binds iron and is admitted into fast growing cancer cells needing iron. Added to the surface of $nTiO_2$.
Tc (Titanocene)	A chemodrug. Additionally it can produces toxic free radicals when activated by light and $nTiO_2$. It attaches to Tf, substituting for iron.
nTiO2-Tf-Tc	A nanoparticle of TiO_2 coated with Tf containing Tc.

How It Works

Schematically, the whole process that occurs within a cancer cell is:

FDG → UV-Blue light → Excites nTiO₂-Tf-Tc → Toxins → Kills Cancer.

The concept is called CRIT (Cherenkov Radiation Induced Therapy). It is a generic cancer therapy and not specifically designed for prostate cancer. The cancer that researchers have tested it in is aggressive human fibrosarcoma—cell colonies and tumors of same formed by injections into mice.

Fibrosarcoma is a cancer of mesenchymal cells in connective tissue. Prostate cancer is generally a carcinoma of epithelial cells. There are differences. One cannot do everything at once — one step at a time.

A cartoon of the major players in a tumor cell is shown in **Figure 16-1.** The role of all the players and their contribution and action to the therapy will be described below.

The radioactive player is FDG, or (18F)fluorodeoxyglucose. This is an analog of glucose, and like glucose, is taken up by cells with a high metabolic rate

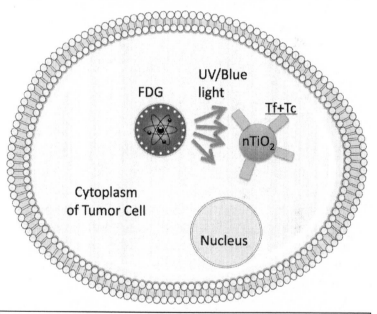

Figure 16-1. A cartoon depiction of the mechanism CRIT therapy. Radioactive (18F)fluorodeoxyglucose (FDG) emits very fast moving positrons (not shown), which because of their faster than light speed, emits Cherenkov light. This strikes a titanium dioxide nanoparticle decorated with Transferin (Tf) and Titanocene (Tc). The light activated nanoparticle produces chemical radicals (not shown) from the contents of the cell. These are toxic to the tumor cell. (For more details see, N Kotagiri et al., Nature Nanotechnology 10, 270-379 (2015).

such as cancer cells. Cancer's high growth rate and aggressiveness is here taken to our advantage. The radionuclide is ^{18}F, a radioactive isotope of fluorine. Fluorine in its stable non-radioactive state is ^{19}F. When it decays, the reaction is $^{18}F \rightarrow {}^{18}O + \beta^+ + \nu$, fluorine releases a positron (β^+) and a massless neutrino, and fluorine converts to a stable oxygen. The neutrino essentially does not interact with matter and sails off into the universe. The emission of the positron comes off at very high energy (633keV) and is traveling about 0.89c, while the speed of light in tissue is about 0.71c. The positron is sailing though tissue faster than the local the speed of light. This produces a "photonic or light boom" and emits Cherenkov radiation in the ultraviolet and blue wavelengths (250-600 nm). For reference, blue light has a wavelength of about 475nm and a black light is about 400nm. This is the light source we require that is inside the body, and preferentially lighting up cancer cells.

FDG is made to serve routinely in cancer imaging using the resulting gamma-radiation. The positron does not travel far since it is antimatter. Antimatter is annihilated when it contacts matter (e.g. us). The reaction, $\beta^+ + e^- \rightarrow 2$ gamma, occurs where both the positron and an electron disappear, poof, and convert their mass into a high energy ($E=mc^2$) form of electromagnetic gamma radiation similar to x-rays. The two gamma rays pass through the body and are routinely used to image tumors. To conserve momentum, one gamma ray goes one way (say North) while the other goes 180 degrees the other way (South). By keeping track of many such events, and drawing lines connecting north with south and east with west and many similar constructs, the location (image) of the tumor is identified within the patient. This is the physics behind a fluoride PET/CT (Positron emission tomography/Computer tomography) scan. Hospitals and clinics do them all the time. They just never see, or use, the Cherenkov radiation lighting up cells.

We now having a "glowing" cancer cell deep within the body. We use this to activate a titanium dioxide (TiO_2) nanoparticle. TiO_2 is a crystalline solid semiconductor and is a bit of a 21st century wonder material. It was initially ignored by the semiconductor industry because wide bandgap means it cannot get electrons to flow by temperature effects and it can only absorb shorter wavelengths of visible light (blue-UV). This property does not make it useful for your computer, but it is useful for certain solar cell applications, hydrogen production from sunlight, and catalytic applications to transfer electrons to chemicals in solution with light. It is that last application, transferring electrons to chemicals that will be useful here. More on that shortly.

We have to get the TiO_2 in the body and into cancer cells, so nanoparticles are used (nTiO2). The National Nanotechnology Initiative started by President Clinton, and supported by President G.W. Bush gave a research push to nano-science (the science of the small). Chemists and physicists were excited about this, but also scratched their heads about the "discovery of nanoscience" by government, as many scientists have been doing nano-science for decades. The word "nano" refers to a nanometer (nm), which is a length measurement of 10^{-9} meters, or a billionth of a meter (a meter is around 1 yard). We require nanoparticles in this application so that they can enter cancer cells within the body. The size of the nTiO2 used is 18nm in diameter, while a cell is around 20,000nm (20μm); clearly $nTiO_2$ is much smaller than a cell. An $nTiO_2$ particle is sort of a giant semiconductor-catalytic molecule. The $nTiO_2$ absorbs light in the 275–390 nm wavelength range, nicely matching the 250-600 nm Cherenkov radiation from FDG.

Why choose TiO_2 for the nanoparticle? As just discussed, its light absorption matches the wavelength of the FDG Cherenkov radiation. But there is a more important reason. That is its ability to transfer electrons to (or from) molecules from (or to) the TiO_2 surface. Light absorbed by a semiconductor elevates an electron to a high energy "conducting" state, leaving behind a missing electron in a "hole." The reaction is light → e- + h$^+$. (A light-emitting diode, like your LED TV, or the somewhat expensive LED lighting bulbs, is the process run backwards, e- + h^+ → light.) The conducting electron or hole, find their way to the TiO_2 surface and can hop onto molecules. This produces reactive oxidative species, or free radicals, which are harmful to cells. One takes vitamin C or other antioxidants to avoid this effect (which occurs naturally at low levels) and which damages healthy tissue. Here we produce radicals only where there is $nTiO_2$ struck by light. If they are in cancer cells, and there is light, we damage the cancer cells. The radicals formed are neutral hydroxyl OH, and superoxide O_2-. Normally hydroxyl molecules are negative, OH-, and normally O_2, an oxygen molecule, is neutral.

But $nTiO_2$ must be dressed up so that cancer cells take it in. Cancer cells are fast growing and require extra nutrients and building material. One necessary element is iron. Iron is shuttled around in the body by a protein called transferrin (Tf). Like the androgen receptor ligand binding pocket, there is a pocket on transferrin for iron. Transferrin proteins are coated on the surface of the $nTiO_2$ particle to produce $nTiO_2$-Tf. Cells take up transferrin protein by transferrin receptors on the cell's surface. Receptors bind to the transferrin protein and swallow up the transferrin and $nTiO_2$ in a process called endocytosis (roughly translated as going inside a cell). The process has again taken advantage of the extreme "hunger" of cancer tumor cells.

Adhering transferrin to $nTiO_2$ to produce $nTiO_2$-Tf is a trick to coax cancer cells to take in the $nTiO_2$ particles. But it allows yet another mechanism to make the nanoparticle more toxic. A chemo drug is adhered to the Tf, which itself is adhered to the $nTiO_2$. The chemo-drug used is Titanocene (Tc), which curiously also has a titanium atom as a central atom in its structure and gives the molecule its name. The final fully dressed nanoparticle is $nTiO_2$-Tf-Tc. Titanocene binds to Tf in the same pocket that Tf uses to binds iron. What a great trick—use Tf to induce the cell to take in the nanoparticle of TiO_2, but do not give it the iron it wants and instead substitute a toxin producing agent. One can imagine adding any number of extra cytotoxins by having them bind to transferrin, but titanocene was chosen because an electron transfer process with $nTiO_2$ too can activate it. In this case it produces additional radicals; $nTiO_2$ when acted on by light breaks up the titanocene into radicals, which interact with molecules in the cell and produce damage of cell contents. This is in addition to it chemo-drug effects.

Some Considerations

The CRIT protocol uses Cherenkov radiation from a well-researched imaging agent (FDG), which is taken up predominantly, but not exclusively, by highly metabolic glucose hungry cancer cells. nTiO2-Tf-Tc nanoparticles are also taken up predominantly, but not exclusively, by fast dividing iron resource seeking cancer cells because of the Tf protein which is normally an iron carrier. The visible and near visible light radiation within the cancer cells interacts with the nTiO2-Tf-Tc nanoparticles and produces chemical radicals that are anxious to interact with normal chemical bonds nearby. This can cause damage (such as cleavage) of molecules, enough of which signals cell death.

A major issue concerning transfer to humans is that both FDG and nanoparticle are not exclusively taken up by cancer cells. To a lesser degree healthy cells engulf them also. But the design here requires "two-to-tango." Both species, FDG and nanoparticles, must be in the same cell at the same time. That is the advantage of having the electron transfer reactions to be driven by light. The two-to-tango hope is that since cancer cells are greedy for both, only cancer cells will be greedy enough to engulf both.

Another curious feature of this protocol is that the light is on in the cancer cells for only a few hours. The half-life of 18F is about 110 minutes. So in about 12 hours, only about 1/64'th of the radiation remains. The damage is done quickly, and does not linger. The damaged cells may linger, but not the damage inducing radiation.

The use of Cherenkov radiation within cells is an unusual way to make cells light up. At first blush, it appears to be a complicated way to produce light. But in fact it is a

258

relatively easy way. It comes for free from a radionuclide that is used routinely for imaging, so presumably its toxicity profile and adverse effects are well known. It has the advantage that its half-life is short and is quickly removed from the patient. The Cherenkov radiation is nicely tuned to TiO_2 absorption, which is a well-studied electron transfer material, and in the absence of light is inert within the body. One can imagine other ways to accomplish what this protocol does, perhaps using light production from a chemical reaction like that used by a lightning-bug. Or making the process more selective of cancer cells by using an antibody similar to what the immune system does to identify cancerous cells. But research in this direction is off to an interesting start with the Washington University work.

Does It Work?
Experiments in Cells

The cells used are human fibrosarcoma cells, specifically a cell line called HT1080. Although not prostate cancer cells, at this early stage it is a proof-of-principle that is being established, not a refinement of a clinical therapy. With cells in a glass dish, one can ask very basic questions and get answers.

The first issue is to truly establish that $nTiO_2$-Tf actually goes into the cells, and does not just adhere to the outside or worse, never actually get near cells. An electron microscope can image cells with extraordinary detail and images clearly show that the $nTiO_2$-Tf particles enter the cells (endocytosis) and are not just nearby or at the surface. This is the desired design feature in that inside they can do real damage. To check that Tf is the agent allowing entry, endocytosis of $nTiO_2$-Tf is stopped by simply adding a significant amount of free floating halo-Tf. Halo-Tf is Tf but with an iron attached. That is the true goal of Tf and the Tf receptor—to admit iron into the cell. The halo-Tf competes with the $nTiO_2$-Tf for admission and the halo-Tf crowds it out. This shows that the Tf receptor process of admission of the nTiO$_2$-Tf is the correct interpretation. Tf is the admission ticket for nTiO$_2$ to enter the cell.

The real test is cell viability, or rather lack of viability, when the cell is treated with nTiO$_2$-Tf-Tc and Cherenkov radiation. Cherenkov radiation is supplied by either of two sources: ^{64}Cu or ^{18}F. ^{64}Cu is similar to ^{18}F but has a longer half-life of 12.7 hours. Cells exposed to nTiO$_2$-Tf-Tc and either ^{64}Cu or ^{18}F reduce their viability by about 80% compared to untreated cells. It is also found that the treated cells had a high amount of damaged DNA which correlated nicely with their reduced viability. The protocol does indeed kill cells. It's not 100%, but optimization of cells in a Petri dish is not the highest priority. Let's get on with living models.

Experiments in Mice

The true story and the power of the method come from experiments in mice. Mice were administered HT1080 cancer cells and tumors developed and in 2-3 weeks would grow to very large size. The game plan is to administer CRIT (Cherenkov radiation induced therapy) to reduce tumor growth and prolong life, or for the tumors to go into remission and disappear. Two strategies are used. The first is to inject the tumor directly with the nanoparticle therapy and the second is to administer the therapy intravenously and have the therapy find the tumor cells themselves via the blood stream. The latter is of course the more useful for human intervention, but even the first is a possibly for certain tumors.

Injection directly into tumors lessens the possibility of toxicity to other organs since the therapy is localized. To ensure that the nTiO$_2$ particles do not transport throughout the body they used nTiO$_2$-PEGS. PEGS? That is a common harmless chemical (polyethylene glycol), often found in laxatives, which is used to decorate nano-objects because of its ability to attach to objects through a process weirdly called Pegylation. TiO$_2$-PEGS does not enter cells like TiO$_2$-Tf does and does not diffuse away as rapidly. Also ^{64}Cu was used as the light supplying Cherenkov radiation source. This experiment is relying on the production of radicals in the vicinity of the tumor cells to cause death.

The results are amazing. After two weeks, untreated tumors, or tumors treated with suboptimal combinations of therapeutic ingredients, increased in volume by 2-4 times, while the treated mice had completely eliminated their tumors. Completely! The tumor exponential decay kinetics were about 40% every three days. Thus direct application of the CRIT protocol to the tumor of a CRIT cocktail kills cells in proximity—cancer cells and otherwise. This has some of the characteristics of radiation therapy, and needs to be applied to a location where the tumor is known to exist with an injection.

The other method is systemic. The CRIT ingredients are injected and both the nanoparticle and radiation source must make a beeline to the tumor and interact within the tumor. The nanoparticle is admitted into the tumor because of the Tf attachment. The radiation source ^{18}F enters the tumor because of the high demand of glucose in tumor cells. It is only when the two are paired that there is the desired reaction. One without the other does not produce CRIT. But nevertheless, some nanoparticles will find their way into other tissue besides tumors and some FDG does as well.

The way it would work in practice is to first inject the nanoparticles and let them settle into the tumor cells of the body. They will stay there for a longer period compared to the time radiation is applied. When ready, then a Cherenkov radiation source such as FDG is injected into the patient. The half-life of FDG is less than 2 hours, so within a few hours the major tumor killing is over. The details of this strategy in humans is not known since no human has undergone this treatment. Phase-I clinical trials would first need to be carried out to assess acceptable dosages. But there are several knobs that can be adjusted. The FDG injection can be repeated say the next day, and another tumor killing session will occur. Or ^{64}Cu can be used which has a half-life 12.7 hours so the tumor killing time can be extended in one session. Or other beta emitters can be used that produce much higher energy particles and hence much more intense Cherenkov radiation.

In an exciting set of experiments, the distribution of nanoparticles can be seen within a mouse. What is being sought is the answer to the question, "How much of nTiO$_2$ goes to tumors and how much goes to other sensitive organs like liver, kidney, brain, bladder heart, blood and so on?" Just how selective is nTiO$_2$ to tumor cells? It is possible to image, with light, inside a whole small animal (mouse).

The light is near infrared radiation. Near infrared is at the very red end of the visible spectrum and goes into the region that our eyes cannot detect. We can detect it as heat, and heat lamps or hot coals produce near IR. But near IR, in the 680-800nm wavelength range is able to be transmitted through tissue (unlike visible light), at least for tissue thicknesses in mice. The way to do this is to add a fluorescent dye to Tf, here called Tf-dye, so that it absorbs light at one wavelength and emits it very shortly thereafter at a slightly longer wavelength. The dye being used absorbs near a wavelength of 680nm and emits at 700-720nm. A whole-animal imager shines 685nm light into the animal, and it takes an image (a kind of photograph) of where the animal "glows" from the fluorescence at 720nm. Either Tf-dye alone or nTiO$_2$-Tf-dye is injected into the tail of the mouse, and an image is taken the next day. Tf-dye by itself (without TiO$_2$) lights up the tumors but there are some other organs that are quite apparent including lung, kidney, liver and blood. The blood lighting up is a result of simply circulating Tf-dye. For the item of interest, nTiO$_2$-Tf-dye, it is the tumor and lungs that shine brightly. The main results are nTiO$_2$-Tf-dye is absorbed by tumors the most, which we assign 100 points, lungs absorb about 25 points, liver and kidney about 10 points, heart and spleen less than 10 points, and so on. Fortunately, the brain received very little, even though nanoparticles of TiO$_2$ do cross the blood brain barrier. The conclusion of all this is that tumors, far and away, endocytose more nTiO$_2$-Tf than other organs, but other organs do absorb a significant amount as well, especially the lungs. This could be problematic. Of course $nTiO_2$-Tf is unlikely to cause any harm if it is there by itself—it needs FDG to produce light to produce radicals to cause damage.

Let's get to the meat—how does the CRIT measure up in preventing the tumor from growing or growing so fast, and preventing the death of mice with tumors? Tumor growth (as measured by tumor volume) with $nTiO_2$-Tf-Tc and FDG was about one eighth the rate it was for untreated mice. Mice treated with nTiO2-Tf, which is without the extra killing power of Tc, also did far better than untreated mice. But it had around a three-fold increase of tumor progression compared to $nTiO_2$-Tf-Tc treated mice. The Tc addition is a major player in the treatment. More advances like this will further improve results. If we leave out the nanoparticle itself, and just treat with Tf-Tc, the growth rate is about twice that of $nTiO_2$-Tf-Tc. Not bad, but overall $nTiO_2$-Tf-Tc produced the superior results. But the tumors still grew. That is the worrisome part. Like many cancer treatments, they buy time. But slowing down the growth rate by 8 (or more) is no small feat. One can hope (and pray) that some additional tweaks will result in a negative growth rate (that is, shrinkage) as was seen in the cell culture experiments.

Survival is the end game—What were the survival results of the mouse model just mentioned? The survival results in mice depended quite a bit on the dosage of the FDG. Mice were in groups of 6. In the untreated group, the first mouse died after about 10 days and all were dead in less than 20 days. For the $nTiO_2$-Tf-Tc with FDG group (high concentration FDG) the first mouse died around 45 days and all were dead at 53 days. This is quite an improvement. Using just Tc-Tf or nTiO2-Tf (without Tc), and of course with FDG, gave intermediate results between untreated and optimally treated. Again the lesson is that including all elements in the therapy produced superior results —results suffer if something is left out. Reducing the dosage of FDG reduced the survival time, and very low dosages produced results similar to untreated mice. There still is the problem that the mice did die, even with optimal therapy and high dosage of FDG, after just about 50 days.

Onward!

This discussion gives an example of things to come. Clearly CRIT is not yet ready for prime time, but these experiments show potential by working on a general cancer therapy, and then hopefully fine-tuning them for specific cancers like prostate cancer. A further improvement that could be made is to add yet a third ingredient to the nanoparticles. Currently one ingredient causes the nanoparticles to enter the cell, a second ingredient allows the nanoparticles to be more potent. We can imagine a third ingredient that might keep the nanoparticles inside the cancer cell for an extended period of time, although it is not clear how long they stay inside the cell. This would allow us to add the radiative component (FDG) multiple times at later dates and still have killing power. In the interim, we can imagine that nanoparticles have been cleared out of other non-cancerous cells so that the toxicity to other organs is minimized. How could this possibly be achieved? One can imagine nanoparticles with an antibody that adheres to the inside of a PCa cell, such as adhering to the androgen receptor. Is this enough to keep the nanoparticle inside the prostate cancer cell? Of course we don't know the answer to that, but ideas along this line can be pursued to keep nanoparticles inside prostate cancer cells while they slowly are released or degrade from other cells. This is only one idea. Your homework assignment is to think of other ideas, perhaps targeting prostate cancer *stem* cells specifically. It is only by some new ideas are we going to move forward.

References

Breaking the depth dependency of phototherapy with Cerenkov radiation and low-radiance responsive nanophotosensitizers, N Kotagiri, GP Sudlow, WJ Akers and S Achilefu, Nature Nanotechnology 10, 270-379 (2015).

Chapter 17

Heading Off Trouble Just In Time: A Look to The Future With Bromodomain Inhibitors.

We must use time as a tool, not as a crutch. John F. Kennedy

We now peek into the future for ways we can interfere with the androgen receptor. The androgen receptor (AR) is the major target for prostate cancer therapy. Androgens like testosterone or DHT bind to the receptor within the prostate cancer cell, which activate the AR to cross into the cell's nucleus. There it finds DNA that it binds to. DNA contains genes and the AR kicks these genes into being expressed, causing the cells to proliferate. Most strategies to halt this sequence of events occur at the front end of the process. Androgen blockade, androgen biosynthesis disruption, and antagonists of the AR all work at the front end before the AR gets anywhere near the DNA located within the cell nucleus.

There is a class of drugs called "BET inhibitors" (or bromodomain inhibitors) that work at the back end of the process. When the AR is activated it binds to DNA to "pull the trigger" to begin the process of transcribing DNA to express genes. BET inhibitors stop the activated AR from binding to the DNA. It is a just-in-time therapy. Thus it is complementary to other androgen interference therapies.

A multi-center team centered at the University of Michigan reported in June 2014 that a small molecule with the enigmatic name JQ1 inhibits AR binding to DNA. This work was done in test tubes and mice, so it is far from being a therapy for humans. It is something for the future — hopefully not the too distant future. Another such molecule is I-BET762, but it has not been tested as extensively. The trick to this strategy is that the AR does not bind directly to

DNA, but rather binds to another molecule BRD4 that binds to DNA. There is kind of AR-BRD4-DNA sandwich stack formed. As usual, biology is not so simple. But this added complexity may be used to our benefit. The finding of the U. Michigan work is that the JQ1 inhibitor is effective in inhibiting the linking of the AR with BRD4. BRD4 plays a role in promoting the expression of genes. The net effect is that the recruitment of the AR to sections of DNA for translation is disrupted.

This means that after all our other androgen receptor interventions have failed, we may still be able to halt the action of the androgen receptor and stop it from promoting the expression of AR-activated genes within the PCa cell.

The Players In This Game

Our star target is BRD4, a protein that is a member of the BET family. (See **Table 16-1** for a short description of the players used in this strategy.) BRD4 helps to recruit the necessary machinery to DNA so that transcription can occur. One of the key machines is RNA polymerase (RNA Pol II) that reads the DNA and transcribes it to RNA. BRD4 helps to assemble other factors so this process can occur. The DNA is in the form of chromatin, which includes a coiled up form of DNA that saves space. The BET family of proteins contains regions, called domains, which bind to chromatin. Those domains are bromodomains. The BET inhibitor, JQ1, binds to a pocket in the so-called bromodomain of BRD4, which results in removing BRD4 from chromatin and also in the removal of RNA Pol II. Most cancer cells express BET proteins, but it not clear if BET inhibitors will disrupt all translation, even in healthy cells.

Table 16-1. The players	Function
JQ1 (and I-BET762)	Small molecule drugs that inhibit the binding of the androgen receptor and BRD4. Inhibition reduces growth and proliferation of cancer cells that are signaled for growth by the androgen receptor.
BET	Family of **B**romodomain and **E**xtra**T**erminal domain proteins. They are DNA (Chromatin) readers. The bromodomain attaches to histones that form a DNA/histone complex called DNA chromatin.
BRD2,3,4,T	BET proteins in humans.
BRD4	The specific BET protein studied here.
Histones	A positively charged protein that winds up the negatively charged DNA. Very long DNA is tightly wound up to fit inside the cell nucleus.
ERG, protein and its gene.	**ETS-regulated g**ene. A transcription factor/regulator. ERG is a member of the erythroblast transformation (ETS) family of genes. ERG is an oncogene. ETS genes play a role in cell proliferation, differentiation, angiogenesis, inflammation and apoptosis and in chromosomal translocations.
Fusion protein/gene	A mutation of the genome where two different DNA genes are fused together resulting in a fused protein upon expression of that gene.
TMPRSS2-ERG	A common prostate cancer fusion protein, especially in CRPC. ERG plays a role in chromosomal translocations. TMPRSS2 is Transmembrane protease, serine 2.
VCaP	An example of a cell line of human cancer. Often it is infused into mice (called a xenograft) to produce tumors in mice for study.

How It Works

Figure 17-1 summarizes the story so far. If these front-end strategies fail (androgen blockade, Enzalutamide, Abiraterone), the AR crosses the cell nuclear membrane as a dimer (AR-AR or AR_2 complex) and enters the inner sanctum of the cell containing DNA. Now we must rely on a

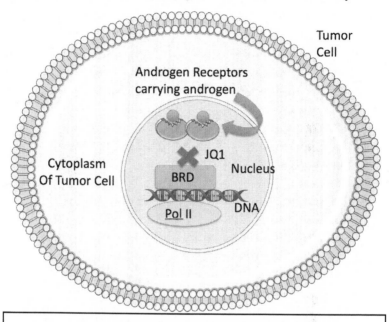

Figure 17-1. Schematic of AR inhibition at the back-end with JQ1. The androgen receptors (ARs) activated by androgen have crossed into the nucleus and seek to form a complex with a Bromodomain protein (BRD) bound to DNA. JQ1 binds to BRD preventing the completion of the full complex and the expression of AR-sensitive genes on the DNA. (More details can be found at: IA Asangani et al., Nature 510, 278-282 (2014).)

back-end, or just-in-time strategy. The bromodomain inhibitor JQ1 binds to BRD4 so that it blocks the formation of the AR_2-BRD4-RNA(Pol II) complex. No complex—no transcription of DNA to RNA and translation from RNA to protein. That's what we want. We do not want our PCa cell expressing the AR dependent genes in the DNA.

The Experiments

The initial experiments (U. Michigan, Ann Arbor) to validate the action of JQ1 were performed on PCa in test tubes, not humans. There are "miles to go before we sleep." Human PCa cells are grown in a cell incubator with growth medium, then torn apart and examined for the proteins that they express using a technique called a Western blot. It is an extension of gel electrophoresis, and is fairly easy to perform. Five different PCa cell lines are used and we just mention one of them, VCaP. This cell line expresses the androgen receptor—this cell line originated from a metastatic site on the vertebrae of a 59-year PCa patient. The patient was castrate resistant. However the cell line is *partially* responsive to hormone deprivation (castration). This cell line expresses the usual proteins; AR, PSA and PAP. Cells also express the mutations of TMPRSS2-ERG and an amplification (excess) of the AR gene.

The cells were grown in different concentrations of JQ1 to see if the drug affects AR, PSA or ERG protein expression. The AR concentration was unaffected, meaning the cells are happily producing androgen receptors. These expressed ARs are anxious to cause the cell to produce PSA and ERG and other proteins causing the prostate cells to grow and proliferate. But the magic is that PSA and ERG protein expression was attenuated. The concentration at which JQ1 inhibited by 50%, the so-called IC50 concentration, was 50nM (nanoMolar). At around a concentration of 500nM both PSA and ERG protein levels were significantly decreased compared to non-treated cells. These data show that the number of AR proteins expressed is unaffected, but the genes expressed by action of the AR are being reduced by JQ1. A great sign!

There is a way to "see" the AR bind to the DNA. This measurement comes from a ChIP-seq experiment (**Ch**romatin **I**mmuno**P**recipitation plus **seq**uencing). It gives a kind of chemical "snapshot" of what is binding to DNA in the act of expressing genes. The basic idea is to remove the DNA from the cells with the chromatin and proteins attached to it, break it up into small pieces, and then grab the pieces that contain protein by passing the sample over appropriate attaching antibodies. Many different antibodies are used, each one selecting for a specific protein bit. Finally the DNA is sequenced, that is its code is read, so that we know what part of the DNA and which gene that protein is adhering to. The protein of interest in these experiments is the androgen receptor. The technique goes back to 2007 and is one of the fairly new tools in the biotechnology toolbox.

What is done here is to compare how often we find the AR binding to DNA under different conditions. Of course we do not want the AR to bind and are looking for conditions where AR binding is reduced. If we stop AR binding, we will halt (hopefully) the progression of the disease. Experiments were made on VCaP cells grown with (A) No Dihydrotestosterone (DHT, a powerful androgen), (B) DHT alone, (C) DHT plus JQ1, and for comparison (D) DHT plus MDV3100 (Enzalutamide) and (E) DHT plus Bicalutamide (Casodex).

The results are shown in **Table 16-2** and are for the AR located anywhere on the genome (DNA). The table shows that with DHT without any inhibitors gives the largest number of ARs bound to DNA.

Table 16-2. ChIP-seq results on VCaP cells	
Treatment of cells	Peak signal (Relative units)
DHT	1.00
DHT + bicalutamide	0.64
DHT + JQ1	0.46
DHT + MDV3100	0.38
Placebo (No DHT)	0.25

We set this peak signal arbitrarily to 1.00, so that comparisons can be easily made. Bicalutamide reduces the peak to 0.64. One sees that JQ1 is preventing AR binding to DNA not as well as MDV3100, but it is not far off. The best results occur if there is no DHT at all, something similar to androgen deprivation therapy. Of course you are wondering about placebo (no DHT) + JQ1. So am I.

In reflecting on these results, keep in mind that this is for one strain of cancer cell (VCaP). Also, the ChIP-seq technique has many variables so that we should view these results as a gross picture of what is occurring. But the gross result is that JQ1 appears to have a positive effect of inhibiting binding of the AR to PCa cells that is expected to result in slowing down disease progression.

Next we need to determine if it works in (i) mice, in (ii) humans, and (iii) is it safe? The science is still at (i), mice. Moving forward requires placing one foot in front of the other. Let's hope we do not need 10 years to move past (ii) and (iii). But for now we have to be content looking at the results in mice. VCaP cells were implanted subcutaneously into mice and allowed to grow into a tumor. The tumors were allowed to grow until they reached a size of $100mm^3$ (about 0.6cm in diameter). At this stage, they were given (5 days a week) either a placebo, MDV3100 or JQ1. After 30 days the tumors had grown on average to $720mm^3$ for the placebo group, $560mm^3$ for the MDV3100 group, and $270mm^3$ for the JQ1 group. In these experiments both MDV3100 and JQ1 both retarded (but not halted) the growth of mouse PCa tumors. But it is clear JQ1 significantly slowed down tumor growth, even far better than MDV3100. As a side effect, JQ1 reduced the size of the testes of the mice. Of all things.

VCaP came from a human patient that was castrate resistant. However in mice, there is some androgen sensitivity. In another set of experiments, mice were subcutaneously implanted with VCaP cells, which were allowed to grow until they reached a volume of $200mm^3$. At this time the mouse was castrated and the tumor receded, until after 2 weeks or so it was back to about $200mm^3$. The PCa is now castration resistant. Now we compare untreated mice (placebo) to mice that received JQ1 for a month. The tumors have grown in the untreated mice by an additional 560mm^3 while tumors grew an additional 220mm^3 in the JQ1 treated mice. The growth rate of the JQ1 treated mice is less than 40% that of the untreated mice.

MDV3100 has a tendency to cause metastases. This is of course a very big deal, especially for patients who have localized prostate cancer. Xenograft experiments were carried out to confirm this in mice and to compare it with JQ1. VCaP cells were injected into mice and tumors were formed. Three distant sites were checked for metastases in these mice, the femur, liver and spleen. Indeed evidence was found that mice treated with MDV3100 had developed metastases. Similar experiments with JQ1 did not show metastases.

Conclusion

The research on BET inhibitors is in its early stages, but it gives us a glimpse of how therapies are tested and what the future holds. Moving this treatment from the laboratory to clinical trials will hopefully follow, but there is no way of knowing what kind of side effects may await, and how effective it truly is in humans. BET inhibitors are well tolerated in mice, do not enhance metastases, and inhibit the growth of PCa in mice. These are some very positive signs with JQ1. However, it does not appear to be a wonder drug, but rather an evolutionary development. Tumors still grow and the AR can still bind. But this direction of research has the potential to extend life in CRPC patients. Let's move ahead full speed.

References

Therapeutic targeting of BET bromodomain proteins in castrate resistant prostate cancer, IA Asangani, VL Dommeti, X Wang, R. Malik, M. Ceislik, R. yang, J Escara-Wilke, K Wilder-Romans, S Dhanireddy, C Engelke, MK Iyer, X jingle, Y-M WU, X cao, ZS Qin, S Wang, FY Feng, and AM Chinnaiyan, Nature 510, 278-282 (2014).

Chapter 18

Concluding With Trouble

Ocian in view! O! the joy
Captain William Clark, Journal, November 1805

Lewis and Clark completed their expedition to the Pacific, and from the above you can feel the excitement of Captain Clark. We are at the end of our expedition but not at the end of our journey. Even over the last 5 years science has made a very positive impact on understanding and treating advanced prostate cancer. But the scientific journey has not yet made it to the "ocian" to produce a durable cure. But we are thankful for the progress made and hope the advances continue at an even accelerated rate.

One thing for sure, being diagnosed with advance prostate cancer does change your world and your worldview. When you are young, you believe you are invincible, then at middle age you become more cautious but believe bad things only happen to others, then when you get older you find out it can happen to you too, and ask *why me?* The worldview changes from concern of the unimportant, to concern for only the important. No one can ruin your day. You simply won't let "them." A day is much more important to you than it used to be, and it is to "them." You feel that you have a pocketful of days remaining rather than a deep well full of them, and each day matters. Time to smell the roses and not worry about the bees.

In examining the state of affairs, I've come to develop certain opinions. In this closing chapter it is appropriate to mention some improvements I'd like to see concerning PCa research and developments, and suggest some actions. But as Mark Twain lectured "Everybody complains about the weather, but nobody does anything about it." So I'll complain about some of the failings in PCa research and treatment with the hope it will have at least some influence in doing something about it. They are just opinions.

Improvements that I'd like to see:

1. Not more research, better research. We need revolution not evolution.
2. Immunology has been disappointing. Gene engineering needs to be revitalized.
3. Trials need improvement.
4. Metformin. A high quality prospective study needs to be completed.
5. Administer Sipuleucel-T early before castrate resistant. Dump the guidebook.
6. Accelerate genomics so it becomes mainstream, especially concerning circulating tumor cells and AR-V7 splice variants.
7. Costs.

More information to consider:

1. Too much research in this field is asking trivial questions, and then not even truly answering the questions it poses. Plenty of examples come to mind, but in the interest in not embarrassing anyone, I won't specifically mention them. It's a general trend to publish more and often—a recipe for static or at best evolutionary research. Fortunately there are many examples of revolutionary research that move the field forward rapidly. An example is the work by CL Sawyers and coworkers at UCLA in 2004, in a paper entitled "Molecular determinants of resistance of antiandrogen therapy," (Chapter 3), which found how the androgen receptor works and how it is responsive to androgen even when it is "hormone refractory." This work was done at a fully equipped biotechnology laboratory using perhaps a dozen different techniques. But they nailed the questions, and changed how we view androgen therapy. This work directly led to Enzalutamide. Without the knowledge of this work, modern methods for treating CRPC concerning the androgen receptor would not

exist. A couple of advances like this every year will move to where we need to be.

2. Immunotherapy has great promise and we should develop it at full speed. However, there appears too much hype for my tastes. Overall it seems to be giving false hope for PCa, at least for the near term. PD-1 and CTLA-4 checkpoint inhibitors have not yet produced much for PCa. We need to regroup on immunotherapy, at least in PCa. It is a given that it is a difficult problem, but advances in PCa have been torturously slow. Some new insights are needed to treat solid tumors with immunotherapy. The sub-area that is really bothersome is gene engineering. Gene therapy shows great promise, yet there is only one group that has moved significantly on this in PCa. And the technique being used is now out of date. It was known when the trial of 4-5 men started that two signals, not one, are needed to fully activate T-cells. The trial started in 2007, and changed design in 2013. Developments in science are happening too fast for a 10-year trial to be meaningful. There is a special disappointment in this field because it does hold promise for a cure. The difficulty is, on one hand, getting the immune system to break though the microenvironment defenses set up by cancer cells, and, on the other hand, not having the immune system indiscriminately attack the patient.

3. Trials need to be improved. They are very stodgy, have much exclusion, and often are dated. At the end of the day they are designed to prove something to the FDA to get a drug/therapy approval. That's what matters. As an example, those with an aggressive disease and who have taken Docetaxel before castrate resistance, because of its recently proven benefits, are excluded from most trials. I know, as I got Docetaxel early and was turned down from some trials. Trial guidelines were written before the early Docetaxel results were known (2014). But the trials continue on

merrily. It's a fast paced world. Apple would not be
in business if it used technology developed five years
ago, and trials need to be flexible as well.

4. There is a case to be made to completely understand
the usefulness of non-cancer drugs on cancer.
Metformin and statins are poster children for this one.
I cannot determine truly whether metformin is useful
or not. Those that say it is helpful show data that
helps far more than the advanced cancer drugs.
Others say it does nothing. It is a pity that this
question remains so controversial. Getting the
question right is the first thing—does it prevent PCa
(one question) or does it slow down progression in
advanced cases (a second question). We need a final
result, especially for the second question, for I don't
see healthy people taking metformin for a disease
that they probably will not get (chances are 1 in 6).

5. Early Sipuleucel-T (Provenge). When the FDA
approves a drug, it is under certain conditions
(indications). There is a catch-22 with Sipuleucel-T.
The earlier it is given the longer it has to act. But one
cannot get it (under most circumstances) unless one
"achieves" castrate resistance. It is almost a certainty
that metastatic PCa will become castrate resistant—
one year, two years, ... five years. Who knows? But
Sip-T is known to slow progression (not cure it). It
takes longer to reach your final dismal destination if
the first half of your trip is 10 mph than if it is 50
mph. Physicians are usually pretty flexible in
dumping the guidebook. No case is the same and
each case requires a specialized strategy. But costs.
Now that is a different matter. It's hard to take an
expensive drug if insurance won't pay for it. And
they won't pay for it unless it is "indicated."

6. Patients and physicians are generally in the dark
about the genetic progression of a patient's disease.
Sure we see lesions in bone scans and have PSA tests
to monitor prostate cancer activity. But getting

genetic information, using liquid biopsies, and analyzing circulating tumor cells is still not mainstream. A case in point is the AR-V7 splice variant for CRPC. This genomic variant is quite useful to determine the resistance mechanism of both Abiraterone and Enzalutamide.

7. Costs. What can I say on this topic that has not been said before? Drugs are outrageously expensive with a special premium added for being in the USA. The argument one always hears is the high cost of developing a drug and bringing it to market. We all get that. Pharmaceuticals are not charities and are in business to make money. Like changing the weather, I'm afraid I can do nothing to change the $100,000 price tag on some cancer drugs. But I will make this observation. Many of the breakthroughs and development of cancer drugs and therapies are not made by the pharmaceutical companies, but rather by much more humble enterprises like laboratories at universities and institutions. Largely, government or charities fund this exploratory work. The intellectual property is then sold to the pharmaceutical companies, or venture capitalists, to develop it further. An example is the CTLA-4 inhibitor Ipilimumab (Yervoy). One group, led by Jim Allison now at MD Anderson, developed the drug and determined how it works. The drug companies run the marketing and trials—the $100,000+ price tag follows. This puts it out of reach for just about everyone. Its use in PCa is uncertain and insurance companies are unlikely to pay for its use. But as a supplement to immunotherapy, such as Sipuleucel-T, it makes sense. Never mind that Sip-T too has a $100,000+ price tag. Clinical trials are expensive and that is part of the problem of high cost. All in all, the development and marketing process does produce amazing benefits. It is unfortunate that it is a bit like farmers and agribusiness. The farmer grows the oats

for a few cents a pound and it is sold for several dollars as Cheerios by the food manufacturer.

Patients are frustrated, and physicians too are now becoming frustrated as the costs have broken any sense of reasonableness and perhaps morality. The issue was taken up in a plenary speech at the 2015 May/June meeting of ASCO (American Society of Clinical Oncology). In his remarks, reported by the Wall Street Journal, Dr. L. Saltz of Memorial Sloan Kettering Cancer Center stated, "Cancer-drug prices are not related to the value of the drug. ... Prices are based on what has come before and what the seller believes the market will bear." That last comment in particular sounds much like what might happen when an entrepreneur sells freshwater to a shipwrecked sailor. The drug cocktail for melanoma of Nivolumab (Opdivo) and Yervoy (Ipilimumab), inspired Dr. Saltz's comments. The cocktail has proven to have significant benefits for melanoma patients—but there is an expected $295,000 price tag for a 1-year dosage. Yervoy (Ipilimumab, or Ipi) our CTLA-4 inhibitor friend of Chapter 12, itself runs around $130,000. One can certainly see the motivation of Pharma to gain FDA approval of Ipi for prostate cancer. Ka-ching.

Enough improvement suggesting and complaining. The world is not perfect, and prostate cancer therapies are advancing at a decent rate. But the different stakeholders view that rate differently. In the special theory of relativity there is a phenomena of time dilation, where time itself changes due to the relative motion between the two timekeepers. There is a sort of time dilation between PCa patients and researchers. Researchers view events as unfolding rapidly while that same time period for patients is excruciatingly long. Time is ticking for the patients and results are needed yesterday.

Progress is being made. We have a way to go to realize the last word in this book which is the most positive word in the business; I hope some truly revolutionary ideas are developed to speed up advancement so that our prostate cancer Lewis and Clark expedition finds its way to our Pacific "Ocian"—a cure.

Index

exons, 83, 84, 92

F

FDG, 252, 253, 254, 255, 257, 260, 262, 263
fermentation, 156
Finasteride, 31, 68
fluorodeoxyglucose, 252, 253
Flutamide, 56, 58
follicle-stimulating hormone, 27

G

gamma, 125, 243, 245, 250, 254
Gene engineering, 228, 273
Gene profiling, 48
Genotropic, 53
Gleason, 6, 7, 16, 97, 129, 213
glutamide, 31
GM-CSF, 196, 197, 204, 214, 216
Goserelin, 31
Granulocyte-Macrophage Colony Stimulating Factor, 196
growth factors, 108, 156
GTP, 134, 135, 136, 138
Guardian of the Genome, 96, 167, 169
guidelines, 21, 38, 274
Gutman, 24
GVAX, 196, 197, 202, 216

H

hazard ratio, 63, 74, 150, 163, 164, 207
heart disease, 33
HIF1a, 157, 158, 159, 160, 163
HIFs, 157
Huggins, 24, 25, 29, 30, 38
hydroxyapatite, 112, 123
hydroxylase, 71
hypothalamus, 25, 26, 27, 29, 30
hypoxia, 156, 157

I

IC50, 71, 268
IL-2, 236, 238, 240, 243, 245, 246

immune checkpoint inhibitors, 173
immunoglobulins, 179, 187
IMPACT, 159, 205, 206, 207, 208, 217
inhibitor, 31, 61, 70, 71, 152, 157, 158, 159, 160, 161, 162, 163, 167, 170, 193, 196, 265, 267, 276
Interleukin, *187*
Intermediate cells, 102, 103
intracrine, 66, 70
intron, 83, 92
Ipilimumab, 196, 197, 200, 276
isotope, 125, 254

J

Janssen Research and Development, 73
Johns Hopkins, 3, 87
JQ1, 264, 265, 266, 267, 268, 269, 270, 271
Junghans, Richard P., 240, 241, 245, 247, 248

K

kallikrein-3, 54
kinases, *190*
knockdown, 52

L

laparoscopic, 6
Lennon, John, 1
leukocytes, *188*
Leuprolide, 28
Leuprolide Acetate, 31
Ligand, 46
ligand binding domain, 45, 84
LNCaP, 167, 168, 169, 202, 215, 216
Luminal cell, 103, 104
Lupron, 23, 28, 31
lyase, 71
Lymphocytes, 174, 175, 182, 219, 248

Sweeney, Chistopher J., 146, 153

T

Tapeworm, 88
TAX327, 138, 139, 140, 153
taxane, 131, 132, 133, 148, 149, 167
Taxol, 131, 132
T-cell receptor, *180, 185, 186, 189, 194, 224, 229, 230, 233, 234, 238, 239, 240*
T-cells, vi, 173, 174, 175, 176, 183, 184, 185, 186, 187, 190, 192, 194, 195, 198, 202, 203, 211, 214, 219, 220, 222, 224, 226, 227, 228, 229, 230, 232, 234, 235, 236, 238, 239, 240, 241, 242, 243, 244, 245, 246, 247, 248, 274
TCR, *180, 185, 186*
Technetium, 7, 113
thymus, 175, 183, 185
titanium dioxide, 252, 254
Titanocene, 252, 256
TMPRSS2, 60, 95, 266, 268
TP53, 95, 96
transcribe, 41, 42, 49, 54, 78, 83, 97, 222, 265
transfection, 224
transferrin, 256
transgenes, 210
translate, 41, 224
translation, 42, 77, 83, 222
translocate, 44, 54, 141, 142
translocates, 47, 55, 61
transrectal ultrasound (TRUS) guided biopsy, 6
Treg, *174, 185*
TRICOM, 199, 210, 217
tubulin, 133, 134, 135, 136, 138, 141, 143, 153
tumor infiltrating lymphocytes, 220, 221

U

UCLA, 40, 42, 57, 104, 273
University of California Los Angeles, 40

University of California-Davis, 88
University of Michigan, 90, 264
urethra, 2, 7

V

vaccines, 173, 196, 201, 204, 209, 213, 214, 215, 216, 218
Valeant, 205
VCaP cells, 269, 270, 271
VEGF, 156
VITAL-1, 216
VITAL-2, 216

W

Warburg, Otto, 156, 170
Washington University, 251, 258
Watson and Crick, 77
Wilson, E. O., x, xi, 4, 20

X

xenograft, 50, 266
Xgeva, 23, 110, 111, 116
Xofigo, 23, 123, 126
XTANDI, 58

Z

Zoladex, 31
Zoledronic acid, 112, 113, 115, 116, 117, 119, 120, 121, 122

ABOUT THE AUTHOR

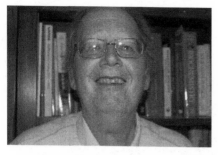 The author is a professional physicist for 35 years, and is a Regents' Professor of Physics, Emeritus, from Arizona State University in Tempe, AZ. He has worked in several areas of physics, mainly theoretical and computational materials physics and biological physics. He is a founding at member of the Center of Biological Physics at ASU, is a Fellow of the American Physical Society, recipient Arizona State University Faculty   Achievement Award – Most Influential Paper (Research) 2007, recipient Distinguished Alumni Award University of Missouri–St. Louis, and twice recipient of teaching awards at ASU. He has authored with students, and collaborators around the world 225 papers in scientific journals such as Science, Proceedings of the National Academy of Science, and Nanotechnology, and his work is highly cited.

He was diagnosed with advance prostate cancer in October of 2013. Since then he has become a prostate cancer "warrior" fighting the disease, facilitates an UsTOO prostate cancer support and education group, and initiated a personal expedition exploring the science of prostate cancer, which he wishes to share here.

You can reach Prof. Sankey at:
TroubledManGland@gmail.com
or visit his website on the science of prostate cancer at
http://TroubledManGland.com